WEIGHT TRAINING WORKOUTS
AND DIET PLAN
THAT WORK

JAMES ORVIS

Ideal Publishing
www.weighttrainingworkouts.com

Note to Readers:
The information in this book is intended to provide a safe, effective nutrition and weight training program. Before starting this or any fitness and exercise program, please consult with your health care provider. The author and publisher are not responsible for any outcomes.

Weight Training Workouts and Diet Plan that Work

Published by:
Ideal Publishing
36695 Pine Bay Drive
Crosslake, MN 56442

Email: james@weighttrainingworkouts.com
Website: www.weighttrainingworkouts.com

ISBN-10: 0-9675188-4-9
ISBN-13: 978-0-9675188-4-8

Layout: Jamie Hukriede
Editing: John Orvis
Cover Design and Illustrations: Kelley Stafne

Printed in the United States of America

Library of Congress Control Number: 2003106611

This book is dedicated to my father-in-law,
Mike Swanson. Miss you.

FITNESS TIP

Drink a big glass of water everyday upon waking. It will do wonders for controlling your appetite plus help build new lean muscle tissue.

Contents

Part I: Your 12 Week Plan To A New You

Contents

Part II: The Best Weight Training Exercises

Contents

Part II: The Best Weight Training Exercises

Contents

Part II: The Best Weight Training Exercises

Getting into shape is actually quite simple.

Here is what you need to know!

Eat wholesome, natural food +75% of the time.
Eat 5-6 small meals each day.
Drink water.
Always eat breakfast.
Have a protein shake 1-3x per day.
Follow a proven weight training program.
Do a cardiovascular activity that you enjoy.

That's it!

Then why doesn't everybody follow this plan?

Because the plan is simple but not easy. In our fast paced society we are constantly confronted with junk food, fast food, new diets, old diets, workout gimmicks and a stream of fads with little time to do any of them.

As many of you have discovered, diets and crazy workouts usually do not work, especially over the long term. Why? Because they either do not work in the first place, or they demand a change in lifestyle so dramatic that you give up and go back to your old habits.

Weight Training Workouts and diet plan that Work will change your life!

It's simple. It's easy. It will get you into shape forever!

Introduction

Here is what works:

1. **YOU NEED TO LIFT WEIGHTS.** Muscle is your engine, your metabolism. It is what burns your calories all day long. But you are constantly losing muscle mass if you do not weight train. Following a proven weight training program will bring back plus add lean, youthful muscles.

2. **YOU NEED CARDIOVASCULAR ACTIVITY.** Your body is meant to move, not sit all day. The solution is very simple. Run, walk your dog, chase your kids or grandkids around, play tennis or go swimming. It does not matter what activity you choose, the big key is to find ones you enjoy, so you will do them!

3. **YOU NEED TO EAT WHOLESOME FOOD 75% OF THE TIME.** If you eat wholesome, natural foods at least seventy-five percent of the time, you will be healthier and lose fat. This allows you to eat whatever you want(within reason), 25% of the time. This is the key to making this plan a lifestyle. Most people want to live a "normal" lifestyle. They want to go out to eat, have some junk food occasionally or maybe a glass of wine. If your fitness program does not allow for these pleasures, most people will fail.

4. **YOU NEED TO EAT 5-6 MEALS PER DAY**. When you eat every 2-3 hours, your metabolism will skyrocket. Its called grazing and this gives your hungry muscles, from working out properly, a constant supply of nutrients. This also keeps your hunger under control so you make smart food choices and do not over eat.

5. **YOU NEED TO DRINK LOTS OF WATER**. Your body is made up of over 70% water. You need it to run properly, look and feel your best. Try to drink at least a gallon of water a day. Have a bottle of water with you at all times. If you feel thirsty, its too late, you are already dehydrated and not running at 100%.

6. **CONSUME 1-3 PROTEIN SHAKES A DAY**. You should ALWAYS have a protein shake after weight training. Within 1 hour of completing your weight training workout your muscles are like a big sponge. They take in twice as many nutrients, twice as fast as normal. When you drink a protein shake it gets into your system fast, so you can use the 1-hour window after weight training to repair and start the muscle building process. This is a major key to fast results with this program. YOU WILL DOUBLE YOUR RESULTS BY USING PROTIEN SHAKES IMMIEDETELY AFTER WORKING OUT!

   You should also use protein shakes (or bars) at other times of the day. They should be considered one of your meals. A high quality shake or bar gives your body everything it needs to build lean muscle and burn fat without excess calories. Breakfast or the last meal of the day are perfect times to use a protein shake or bar.

   If you are looking for maximum fat loss, here is good rule of thumb to live by... *Every other meal should be a protein shake*! It works, they taste great, they are good for you and they will fill you up both mentally and physically.

7. **USE A SPECIAL 5-DAY LOW CARB WEEK**. If you use low carbs timely and precisely, it is one of the greatest tools for losing fat AND gaining lean muscle(instead of losing muscle on many other diets). The secret is; be following a proven weight training program, a healthy food plan and for only 5 days do not eat any carbohydrates. It will have an amazing effect on your body composition. It is quite possible to <u>lose 3-4 pounds of fat</u> in a week plus bust through any plateaus and add rock hard muscle the following week. You will find out exactly what to do in week 4.

That's it!

These 7 simple keys will help you lose weight and be fit for life.

3 Parts of Food

Food is very important to getting into shape and staying in shape.

This is the best way to think about it.

Weight training and cardio, are the stimuli for your body to use food in the best possible way. After you exercise properly, what you eat will determine ongoing and final results of your fitness program.

YOU HAVE TO EXERCISE FIRST FOR YOUR BODY TO USE FOOD WISELY.
If you do not exercise then a lot of what you eat is stored as fat!

Hypothetically, if I was forced to choose between exercising right and eating junk food, or not exercising and eating a perfect, clean diet, I would choose the exercise and cookies.

I say that to make a point on how important weight training and cardio are to being healthy and in shape.

After you work out, what you put into your mouth and when it goes in, will determine how fast your body changes. 75% of the results will happen after you workout. Eat small, wholesome meals every 4 hours and your body will be lean and mean in a short time!

Here is what you need to know about food to be fit and healthy.

There are three basic components of food.

Carbohydrates
Proteins
Fats

To make it simple;
-carbohydrates are for energy
-proteins are for building and maintaining muscle
-fats are for making hormones & are used as energy /stored as future energy.

<u>You need all three to be healthy, fit and ALIVE</u>.

They are not good or bad.

Only bad when taken in the wrong doses and at the wrong time.

NOTE: I do not tell you *exactly* how much food and calories to consume. If you are too concerned with calorie counting, portion size or weighing your food, most people will fail. It is hard, not fun and not necessary.

When you eat wholesome, real foods plus protein shakes at least 75 percent of the time, YOU WILL NOT EAT TOO MUCH! You will be mentally and physically full and satisfied. It works!

3 Parts of Food

Here is how to consume each food part for maximum benefits to your health and waistline.

CARBOHYDRATES (Carbs)

Carbs are everywhere, as you probably know. It is not difficult to find carb foods and it is very easy to overeat on them. They are especially present in our current food culture as refined foods have become popular, abundant, inexpensive and so very convenient. Included are foods like breads, chips, pastries, cookies, ice cream, pastas and candy. JUNK FOOD! They taste great but these simple carb foods are loaded with calories with little good nutritional value.

Complex carbohydrates are what you should be eating most of the time. These are the wholesome natural foods like vegetables, fruits, whole wheats, nuts, beans, brown rice and oatmeal. These will provide a good supply of vitamins, minerals and fiber along with the complex carbs.

Eat approximately 1-2 grams of carbohydrates per body weight per day.

Example: You weigh 200 lbs = 200-400 grams per day.
Carbs have 4 calories per gram = 800-1600 calories per day.

If you are very active or want to add weight, eat more carbs.

PROTEIN

Protein is for building muscle. You find protein mainly in meat, fish, dairy, legumes, eggs, soy, protein shakes and bars.

You should try to include a protein source in every meal. The main reason is that your body only retains protein in your blood, from what you have eaten, for a maximum of 4 hours. After 4 hours your body will need protein to keep doing thousands of bodily processes, so it gets protein from you. If you did not eat some protein...it breaks down your hard earned muscles for the protein! Exactly what you do not want to happen.

To be fit and healthy the key is to eat 5-6 small meals a day, always with a protein source. It's that easy.

Your daily diet should be about 1 gram of protein, per pound of bodyweight.

Example: You weigh 200 lbs = 200 grams per day.
Protein has 4 calories per gram = 800 calories per day.

FAT
Fat is used for thousands of metabolic processes. But for simplicity sake in this book, the fats you eat are used for energy, making hormones and losing fat.

Good fats are found mostly in meat, fish, eggs, dairy, olive oil, avocados, and nuts.

Bad fats are trans-fatty acids and saturated fats, found in a plethora of processed and junk foods, Such as potato chips, deep fried foods and pastries. Too many saturated fats from fatty meats are also undesirable.

Consume about .25% grams of fat per body weight per day.

Example: You weigh 200 lbs = 50 grams per day.
Fat has 9 calories per gram = 450 calories per day.

Eat more fats if you are very active, younger or want to add weight.

12 Food Secrets

In the order of importance!

1. Eat 4-6 small nutritious meals every day.
2. Drink at least one gallon of pure water each day. One of the most important things you can do to make you body run optimally and to keep your appetite under control.
3. Find a protein shake that you like and use it. There are many super brands and tasty flavors . Check the internet or your local health food store. Switching proteins occasionally is a good idea, so your body receives a variety of different nutrients. Mix protein powders with water, milk or juice. Only use juice with the protein shake AFTER weight training. Your muscles need the juice(sugar) for muscle repair.
4. Always eat breakfast within 30 minutes of waking.
5. Eat a majority of your carbohydrates in the first half of the day & before and after weight training. Eat less carbs at night. Do not eat carbs by themselves. Always have a protein or protein & fat source with carbs. This keeps your blood sugar stable.
6. Avoid pasta, white rice and white breads. These 3 "good foods" are loaded with empty processed carbs and calories and you will always eat too much! Many people lose a lot of unwanted weight just by dropping these three foods from their diet.
7. When eating out, order grilled, baked and broiled lean meats and fish, steamed or raw vegetables and salads.
8. Take a good multi-vitamin with breakfast. Take a good multi-mineral before bed.
9. Take 2-5 grams of omega 3 fatty acids every day. Flaxseed oil, walnut oil and fish oils are the best.
10. Buy 100% whole wheat products. If it does not say 100% it can contain as little as 1% whole wheat. Don't be fooled!
11. Buy an oil sprayer and fill with virgin olive oil. Virgin olive oil is a *good fat* that is very beneficial to your health and losing fat. Use it in any cooking method.
12. If you have a craving for your favorite junk food, have a little and move on. "Cheat Meals" are needed and deserved!

Weight Training Basics

The Four Keys

There are many factors to successful weight training. However there are four main keys you must know. Using this knowledge will guarantee maximum results in the least amount of time.

1. Proper Form

The exercises you will perform are described with simple instructions and pictures. Study and practice the exercises with light weights until you become comfortable with the movements. Your form is crucial for maximum results and safety. Follow the exercise technique section as closely as possible. Do not watch other people workout, most are doing it wrong.

2. Intensity

Once you learn proper exercise form, you should put total concentration into every rep of each set. Focus on the muscles you are working. Study and practice the exercises so you know which muscles are being used. Weight training is at least 50 % mental. Learn to concentrate on the muscles you are working, then they will become lean and fat free!

The second part to intensity is very, very important. Do as many repetitions as you can, and then try 2 more, always with good form, of course. *This is called muscle fatigue or muscle failure.* The main reason your body is going to change (lose fat, firm up, add muscle, become stronger and healthier), is because your body believes it has to in order to survive. It is that simple. If you do not challenge your body by trying a couple more reps, it will stay the same. These are called the magic reps. They truly are because they will give you a fit and fabulous body.

Weight Training Basics

The Four Keys

3. Variety

The third principle you must know is variety. Your body needs to be challenged, as in muscle fatigue, but it also is super-adaptable. If you do the same workout, day after day, week after week, you will get diminishing returns with every workout. Little to no results! Even if you are giving your best effort this will happen. Your body learns very quickly the exercises, weights used, reps, and sets. Because it adapts it will use less muscle to perform the exercises. This is exactly what you do not want to happen. You want to keep your body guessing, so it is constantly changing and improving.

4. Consistency

The last principle to successful weight training is that your body needs regular weight training exercise to make improvements in your health and physical appearance. This does not mean you need to workout for hours every day. In fact that is precisely what you do not want to do. Like many people who start an exercise program, you will most likely wear out your body and quit. Consistency means following this book as closely as possible. The proven routines will give you maximum results with a commitment of only an hour or two per week. That's not much time to invest in your health and body. It will be one of the best investments you ever make!

What you really need to know

Barbell (BB)
Long bar usually 4 to 7 feet in length, you hold it with both hands.

Dumbbell (DB)
Short bars about a foot in length, you can hold one in each hand.
Dumbbells come in a variety of designs and sizes.

Repetition (Rep)
Lifting the weight and lowering the weight to the starting point
equals one repetition.

Set
Completing as many repetitions as you can on an exercise equals one set.

Tempo
The speed that you perform the exercise.
For maximum results and safety:

Lift the weight for 1-2 seconds.
This is called the *positive* part of the exercise

Lower the weight for 2-3 seconds.
This is called the *negative* part of the exercise

A slow, controlled tempo makes your muscles do all the work.
A controlled speed is also easier on your joints.

Weight Training Basics

Breathing

Proper breathing is very important and you need to practice and exaggerate your breathing when you first start weight training. *Do not hold your breath!*

Exhale when you lift (*positive part*) the weight.
Inhale when you lower (*negative part*) the weight.

Warming up

Always warm-up before weight training. The best way to warm up is to do approximately five to ten minutes of a cardiovascular activity. Walking, biking or the stair climber all will work nicely. Second, lift light weights, using about 50 percent of the weight you will be using during your workout routine. Warm up on all the exercises you are going to perform during your workout. To function properly, your muscles need the increased blood flow that a warm-up provides. Most people do not warm-up enough. Make sure you do!

When you are ready to give *maximum effort*, begin your workout.

Amount of weight to use on each exercise

Each exercise has a range of weight to choose from in pounds.

The weight is recommended for women.
Men should double the recommended weight.

Always start with the lightest weight suggested!

When the weight is recommended for a dumbbell (DB) exercise, the weight is for each dumbbell.

These are only recommended weights, so you will know where to begin on each exercise especially if you are new to weight training or a particular exercise.

Make sure to increase the weight when it is too light!!

26

Muscle Fibers
Your body is composed of many different kinds of muscle fibers.
The are two main types we are concerned within this book.

1. Endurance Muscle Fibers
   They increase in endurance but do not gain much in size or strength.
   This increase will not assist a lot in burning more calories and fat at
   rest. Endurance muscles respond best to aerobic activity and high
   repetition weight training (more than 20 reps).

2. **Strength Muscle Fibers**
   They become stronger, larger and more abundant with proper weight
   training. This correlates into more calories burned at rest, even when
   you are lying on the sofa! These are the muscle fibers you want to
   target when lifting weights. They respond best to 5-15 repetitions to
   muscle failure.

Muscle Fatigue (Muscle Failure)
You cannot complete one more rep with good form.

Rest Periods
Amount of time you rest between sets.

Spotter
A spotter helps the lifter during the exercise. He or she assists in moving
the weights into the starting position, helps during the lift so more reps
are possible and encourages the lifter to give his or her best effort.

If exercise equipment is not available
Choose a different exercise for the same muscle group.

Try working out at the same time everyday.
It is much easier to stay on course
with a plan and planned time.

12 Secrets in order of importance!

1. **Show Up!** The biggest results you will receive from weight training is to show up. 80% of success in anything you do, is to just do it. You will see incredible results if you follow this program.

2. **Make Every Set Your Best.** Weight training is a sprint. After you are warmed-up, make every set the best you can do. Do not hold back for the next set. It is not a marathon where you pace yourself. That is for a cardiovascular activity. Go to muscle fatigue on each set, and your body will be forced to become lean and fit.

3. **Use The Right Amount of Weight For Your Strength.** Maximum results come from muscle fatigue in the 8-15 rep range. If the weight is too light, and feels light at the beginning of the set & you can do more than 15-20 reps, IT IS TOO LIGHT! You are then doing a cardiovascular activity and not strength training. Use a heavy enough weight for maximum results and increase the weights when needed. Your strength will increase quickly with these workouts.

4. **Drink A Protein Shake Right After Weight Training.** I know this is in the food section but you will <u>double your results</u> from the workouts if you remember to have a shake within 1 hour of completing your workouts. Just do it!

5. **Find A Workout Partner.** A workout partner is one of the best things you can do in your fitness quest. They help you spot, push you during the exercises, make you show up for your workouts and don't allow you to slip on your eating habits. Find one if possible.

Weight Training Basics

6. **Listen To Music You Enjoy.** Listening to music that you like will get you fired up! Music makes exercising more fun. You also become a lot stronger, more focused and willing to do those extra magic reps.

7. **Stretch at the end of your workouts.** <u>Do not</u> stretch at the beginning of your workouts (but always warm up thoroughly with aerobic activity & light weight training). Your muscles need to be warmed up and elastic to stretch safely. You want to stretch after lifting weights.

8. **Don't count reps until you are tired.** You want your muscles to fatigue close to the prescribed number of repetitions laid out in this book. BUT you do not want to make that number all important. It is a reference. Far too many people are only concerned with completing a certain number of reps. Your muscles do not count, they respond to a stress. If you are suppose to do 10 reps and get to 10 reps and can still do more with good form – do them! You can increase the weight on your next set or workout. **Start counting when your muscles become tired**. Tell yourself you are going to do 3 more reps. This is when your body really firms up and turns into a fat burning machine!

12 Secrets in order of importance!

9. **Do cardio on non-weight training days.** For maximum fat loss and muscle gain, do your cardio on your non-lifting days if time permits. This will give your muscles time to recover from weight training and become stronger. If you want to do your cardio on your weight training day, do it *after* lifting weights. Weight training uses a lot of quick energy. The sugar in your body, used for fuel is called glucose and glycogen. After your weight training workout, your body is low on "sugar" and has to use fat for energy. This is what you want to happen when performing your aerobic activity. Do cardio 2-4x per week, 20-45 minutes per session. Make it an activity that you enjoy so you will do it consistently.

10. **Concentrate on the muscles you are targeting.** When you can feel and visualize the muscles you are using during an exercise, you are well on your way to being fit & firm.

11. **Read other fitness books and magazines.** Learn as much as you can on nutrition and exercise. It is a science that is constantly evolving, especially nutrition and supplements.

12. **JUST SHOW UP...IT WORKS.**
    Had to say it again.!!!!!

If you workout at home, consider purchasing a Vertical Leg Press. It is a very cost effective piece of exercise equipment that targets the lower body.

ARE YOU READY!

You are about to start on a life-changing mission. Eating right and exercising properly are two of the most important things you will ever do for living a successful, happy life.

YOUR HEALTH IS YOUR WEALTH —DON'T FORGET IT!

In week 1 you will be easing your body and mind into eating the right way and working out. Again, it is very simple to do and doesn't need to throw your life into chaos. Just a few easy changes to build that body you have always wanted.

FOOD
The food plan is fully set up for you. Follow it as closely as you can. It is a very basic menu. Make it simple, it will still taste great! Change it to fit your life where needed. Be sure to eat wholesome natural foods 75% of the time and always have your protein shake after working out. When you do these two things, you will not overeat, because it is very hard to overeat wholesome foods and protein shakes. You will get results!

Two things to remember.

1. NUMBER OF MEALS. If you are now eating only 2, 3 or 4 meals a day, only add 1 more meal a day in week 1. If you try to go from 2 meals a day to 6 meals a day, your body will revolt and you will quit. You need to ease into the right way to eat. Then in week 2 you

can add 1 more meal a day. Add 1 more meal per week until you are eating the 5-6 meals per day.

2. PROTEIN SHAKES. If you have never used protein shakes before, start out slow. Start with a very small shake after weight training and gradually make it the appropriate size for your weight and goals. Just like eating too many meals right away, consuming to large or too many protein shakes will send your stomach into a tailspin. Shakes have a lot of nutrients that get into your system fast and if you are not used to it, you will get an upset stomach. Ease into them, find the protein that you like, and you will turn into a fat burning machine.

WEIGHT TRAINING
In Week 1 you will be performing Straight Sets.

Straight Sets
- Complete prescribed number of reps on set #1.
- Rest 1-2 minutes.
- Complete second set of the same exercise.
- Rest 1-2 Minutes
- Move on to the next exercise.

Straight Sets are the most basic way to weight train. It allows you to concentrate on using perfect form and taking each set to muscle fatigue. If you are new to weight training or have not lifted weights consistently, do not lift to failure the first week. Choose a weight on each exercise that will allow you to complete the number of reps suggested when the exercise starts to become challenging.

Week 1: Straight Sets

Week 1

- Three weight training workouts.
- Non consecutive days.
Example: Monday-Wednesday-Friday or whatever works for you. Try to have at least one day of rest between weight training workouts. Cardio 2 days. On non-lifting days. 15-30 minutes.
- Total body workouts.
- 8 exercises per workout.
- Two sets per exercise.
- Rest 1-2 minutes between sets.
- 10 repetitions to muscle fatigue. Each exercise will have a prescribed number of reps for the best results. Try to hit muscle fatigue at or around this number. Start with the lightest weight recommended and add more weight if it's too easy and you are completing more reps than suggested.
- Remember – if you are new to weight training, stop before muscle fatigue in the first week of lifting. You can increase the intensity in week 2 and go to muscle failure in week 3.
- Remember - men <u>double</u> the recommended weight.
- **Make sure to warm up for 5-10 minutes with light weights before starting your workouts. You can also do aerobic activity to warm up but ALWAYS include light weight training, using about 50% of your workout weights.**

Week 1 - Monday
Food Menu

Today's Menu	What I ate
1. 2-3 Eggs 2 100% Whole Wheat Toast	
2. Baked Potato Cottage Cheese Turkey Breast	
3. Protein Shake	
4. Handful of Nuts Piece of Fruit	
5. Baked Fish Steamed Vegetables Brown Rice	
6. String Cheese	

Week 1: Straight Sets
Workout 1
-Total Body-

Exercise	Your Goal Reps x Weight		Your Set Reps x Weight	
1. DB Bench Press	10	5-15		
DB Bench Press	10	5-15		
2. DB Curls	10	5-12		
DB Curls	10	5-12		
3. Pullovers	10	5-15		
Pullovers	10	5-15		
4. DB Press	10	3-12		
DB Press	10	3-12		
5. Lat Pulldown*	10	25-50		
Lat Pulldown	10	25-50		
6. Leg Extensions	15	20-40		
Leg Extensions	15	20-40		
7. Leg Press	15	40-75		
Leg Press	15	40-75		
8. Ab Bench Crunch	15	0		
Ab Bench Crunch	15	0		

*Wide Grip

Week 1 - Tuesday
Food Menu

Today's Menu	What I Ate
1. Plain Yogurt with Grapenuts and Fruit	
2. Turkey Sandwich on 100% Whole Wheat Bread Baked Chips	
3. Protein Shake	
4. Celery with Peanut Butter	
5. Grilled Chicken Salad Light Dressing	
6. Protein Bar or Glass of Milk	

Week 1 - Tuesday
Cardio Activity
20-30 Minutes

Week 1 - Wednesday
Food Menu

Today's Menu	What I Ate
1. 2-3 Eggs Baked Potato	
2. Turkey Jerky	
3. Tuna Fish Sandwich on 100% Whole Wheat Bread	
4. Protein Shake	
5. Lean Hamburger Steamed Vegetables	
6. Glass of Milk or Yogurt	

Week 1: Straight Sets
Workout 2
-Total Body-

Exercise	Your Goal Reps x Weight		Your Set Reps x Weight	
1. DB Bench Press	10	5-15		
DB Bench Press	10	5-15		
2. DB Curls	10	5-12		
DB Curls	10	5-12		
3. Pullovers	10	5-15		
Pullovers	10	5-15		
4. DB Press	10	3-12		
DB Press	10	3-12		
5. Lat Pulldown	10	25-50		
Lat Pulldown	10	25-50		
6. Leg Extensions	15	20-40		
Leg Extensions	15	20-40		
7. Leg Press	15	40-75		
Leg Press	15	40-75		
8. Ab Bench Crunch	15	0		
Ab Bench Crunch	15	0		

Week 1 - Thursday
Food Menu

Today's Menu	What I Ate
1. Protein Shake	
2. String Cheese Raw Vegetables	
3. Turkey Wrap	
4. Cup of Cottage Cheese Piece of Fruit	
5. Bowl of Chili Whole Wheat Crackers	
6. Protein Bar or Piece of Deli Turkey/Roast Beef	

Week 1 - Thursday
No Organized Exercise

Week 1 - Friday
Food Menu

Today's Menu	What I Ate
1. Oatmeal with Raisins	
2. Protein Shake	
3. Grilled Chicken Breast Coleslaw	
4. Cottage Cheese Bowl of Fruit	
5. Grilled Steak Salad	
6. Handful of Nuts	

Week 1: Straight Sets
Workout 3
-Total Body-

Exercise	Your Goal Reps x Weight		Your Set Reps x Weight	
1. DB Bench Press	10	5-15		
DB Bench Press	10	5-15		
2. DB Curls	10	5-12		
DB Curls	10	5-12		
3. Pullovers	10	5-15		
Pullovers	10	5-15		
4. DB Press	10	3-12		
DB Press	10	3-12		
5. Lat Pulldown*	10	25-50		
Lat Pulldown	10	25-50		
6. Leg Extensions	15	20-40		
Leg Extensions	15	20-40		
7. Leg Press	15	40-75		
Leg Press	15	40-75		
8. Ab Bench Crunch	15	0		
Ab Bench Crunch	15	0		

*Wide Grip

Week 1 - Saturday
Food Menu

Today's Menu	What I Ate
1. 2-3 eggs Whole Grain English Muffin	
2. Protein Shake	

3. Bowl of Soup
   Side Salad
   Whole Wheat Bread	

4. Apple & Cheese	
5. Broiled Shrimp Steamed Vegetables	
6. Protein Bar	

Week 1 - Saturday
Cardio Activity
20-30 Minutes

Week 1 - Sunday
Food Menu

Today's Menu	What I Ate
1. Waffle & Sugar Free Syrup Turkey Ham	

2. Baked Potato
   Roast Beef
   Cottage Cheese	

3. Grilled Chicken Salad	
4. Fruit & Yogurt	

5. Tuna Fish Sandwich on
   Whole Wheat Bread
   Raw Vegetables	

6. Protein Shake	

Week 1 - Sunday
No Organized Exercise

www.1fast400.com is a great website to buy protein shakes and supplements with real buyer's reviews of their effectiveness.

Week 2: Straight Sets

Did you survive week 1? Pretty easy, right?

The key to success is to ease into it and do it right.

Now you will be performing Straight Sets again with new exercises.

During week 1, you worked on the same 8 exercises each workout. You will now be adding different exercises in week 2. Try to complete 1 extra rep with perfect form. Week 1 started your foundation, now in week 2 you should feel more comfortable with lifting weights.

Week 2

- Three Workouts.
- Non-consecutive days.
- Total Body Workouts.
- 8 exercises per workout.
- 2 sets per exercise.
- Rest 1-2 minutes between sets.
- REMEMBER-
- Make sure to warm up for 5-10 minutes.
- Rep Speed: 1-2 seconds on Positive part of the exercise, 2-3 seconds on the Negative part of the lift.
- Breathing. Exhale on the Positive, Inhale on the Negative. NEVER HOLD YOUR BREATH!

Week 2 - Monday
Food Menu

Today's Menu	What I Ate
1. 2-3 eggs 100% Whole Wheat Toast	
2. Protein Shake	
3. Grilled Chicken Salad	
4. Protein Shake	
5. Baked Fish Brown Rice Steamed Vegetables	
6. String Cheese	

Week 2: Straight Sets
Workout 1
-Total Body-

Exercise	Your Goal		Your Set	
	Reps x	Weight	Reps x	Weight
1. BB Bench Press	10	20-45		
BB Bench Press	10	20-45		
2. BB Curls	10	10-20		
BB Curls	10	10-20		
3. Pullovers	10	5-15		
Pullovers	10	5-15		
4. BB Press	10	10-20		
BB Press	10	10-20		
5. Lat Pulldown*	10	25-50		
Lat Pulldown	10	25-50		
6. Leg Curls	10	15-30		
Leg Curls	10	15-30		
7. DB Squats	15	5-15		
DB Squats	15	5-15		
8. Ball Crunches	15	0		
Ball Crunches	15	0		

*Underhand Grip

Week 2 - Tuesday
Food Menu

Today's Menu	What I Ate
1. Protein Shake	
2. Baked Potato Cottage Cheese Black Olives	
3. Turkey Sandwich Banana	
4. Protein Shake	
5. Grilled Lean Steak Side Salad	
6. Glass of Milk or Yogurt	

Week 2 - Tuesday
Cardio Activity
20-40 Minutes

Week 2 - Wednesday
Food Menu

Today's Menu	What I Ate
1. Protein Shake	
2. Cottage Cheese Bowl of Fruit	
3. Lean Hamburger Baked Chips	
4. Protein Shake	
5. Grilled Chicken Breast Sweet Potato/Yam	
6. Glass of Milk, Yogurt or Nuts	

Week 2: Straight Sets
Workout 2
-Total Body-

Exercise	Your Goal		Your Set	
	Reps x	Weight	Reps x	Weight
1. BB Bench Press	10	20-45		
BB Bench Press	10	20-45		
2. BB Curls	10	10-20		
BB Curls	10	10-20		
3. Pullovers	10	5-15		
Pullovers	10	5-15		
4. BB Press	10	10-20		
BB Press	10	10-20		
5. Lat Pulldown*	10	25-50		
Lat Pulldown	10	25-50		
6. Leg Curls	10	15-30		
Leg Curls	10	15-30		
7. DB Squats	15	5-15		
DB Squats	15	5-15		
8. Ball Crunches	15	0		
Ball Crunches	15	0		

*Underhand Grip

Week 2 - Thursday
Food Menu

Today's Menu	What I Ate
1. Oatmeal made with Milk	
2. Celery W/ Peanut Butter	
3. Protein Shake	
4. String Cheese	
5. Fajitas	
6. Protein Shake	

Week 2 - Thursday
No Organized Exercise

Week 2 - Friday
Food Menu

Today's Menu	What I Ate
1. Omelet Whole Wheat Toast	
2. Protein Shake	
3. Tuna Fish Sandwich Raw Vegetables	
4. Protein Shake	

5. Grilled Chicken
    Brown Rice
    Side Salad	

6. Glass of Milk or Yogurt	

Week 2: Straight Sets
Workout 3
-Total Body-

Exercise	Your Goal		Your Set	
	Reps x	Weight	Reps x	Weight
1. BB Bench Press	10	20-45		
BB Bench Press	10	20-45		
2. BB Curls	10	10-20		
BB Curls	10	10-20		
3. Pullovers	10	5-15		
Pullovers	10	5-15		
4. BB Press	10	10-20		
BB Press	10	10-20		
5. Lat Pulldown*	10	25-50		
Lat Pulldown	10	25-50		
6. Leg Curls	10	15-30		
Leg Curls	10	15-30		
7. DB Squats	15	5-15		
DB Squats	15	5-15		
8. Ball Crunches	15	0		
Ball Crunches	15	0		

*Underhand Grip

Week 2 - Saturday
Food Menu

Today's Menu	What I Ate
1. Protein Shake	
2. Piece of Fruit & Nuts	
3. Grilled Chicken Sandwich Baked Beans	
4. Protein Shake	

5. Grilled Fish
   Steamed Vegetables
   Baked Yam	

6. Jerky	

Week 2 - Saturday
Cardio Activity
20-40 Minutes

Week 2 - Sunday
Food Menu

Today's Menu	What I Ate
1. Roast Beef Baked potato Melted Cheese	
2. Protein Shake	
3. Turkey Sandwich	
4. Protein Shake	
5. Grilled Chicken Brown Rice Side Salad	
6. Yogurt or Protein Bar	

Week 2 - Sunday
Rest

Week 3: Pyramid-up

In Week 3 you will use Pyramid-up workouts. This gives you a simple and effective way to increase your strength, build lean muscle and turn your into a fat burning machine.

Pyramid-up

- Three sets of an exercise.
- Increase the weight each set.
- Lower rep goal each set.
- 2-3 minutes between each set.

Example: Barbell Bench Press

SET 1: 12 reps x 45 lbs.
   ↓ Rest 3 minutes
   Increase the weights

SET 2: 10 reps x 55 lbs.
   ↓ Rest 3 minutes
   Increase the weights

SET 3: 8 reps x 65 lbs.
   ↓ Rest 3 minutes
   Go to the next exercise

You should be aiming for close to muscle fatigue in your 3rd week. When each set starts to become difficult, try 2 more reps. This is when you make the most progress...this is when you BUILD MUSCLE!!!!!!!!!!

Have you found a protein shake you love? There are many great tasting shakes that will make losing weight and building muscle a lot faster and more enjoyable. You will be using 2-3 shakes a day in week 3 so find the right one!

Week 3

- Four workouts.
- 5 exercises per workout.
- 3 sets per exercise.
- 12-10-8 reps.
- Rest 2-3 minutes between sets. When you rest up to three minutes between sets, you reclaim most of your strength. This allows you to perform the maximum amount of reps on your next set.
- Warm up! You should feel like you are ready to give maximum effort on the 1st set of your workout.

Week 3 – Monday
Food Menu

Today's Menu	What I Ate
1. Protein Shake	
2. Celery with Peanut Butter	
3. Grilled Chicken Sandwich	
4. Protein Shake	
5. Turkey Wrap	
6. Protein Shake or Bar	

Week 3: Pyramid-Up
Workout 1
Chest, Shoulders, Triceps

Exercise	Your Goal		Your Set	
	Reps x	Weight	Reps x	Weight
1. Incline DB Bench	12	8-20		
Incline DB Bench	10	8-20		
Incline DB Bench	8	8-20		
2. Incline Flys	12	5-12		
Incline Flys	10	5-12		
Incline Flys	8	5-12		
3. BB Press	12	10-25		
BB Press	10	10-25		
BB Press	8	10-25		
4. Side Raise	12	3-12		
Side Raise	10	3-12		
Side Raise	8	3-12		
5. Pushdowns	12	50-75		
Pushdowns	10	25-50		
Pushdowns	8	8-20		

Week 3 - Tuesday
Food Menu

Today's Menu	What I Ate
1. Protein Shake	

2. Baked Potato
   Cottage Cheese
   Turkey Breast	

3. Yogurt with Fruit	
4. Protein Shake	

5. Lean Steak or Chicken
   Steamed Vegetables
   Whole Wheat Bread	

6. Protein Shake or Bar	

Week 3: Pyramid-Up
Workout 2
-Legs, Abs -

Exercise	Your Goal		Your Set	
	Reps x	Weight	Reps x	Weight
1. BB Squats	12	25-50		
BB Squats	10	25-50		
BB Squats	8	25-50		
2. Leg Press	12	50-100		
Leg Press	10	50-100		
Leg Press	8	50-100		
3. Calf Raises	12	50-100		
Calf Raises	10	50-100		
Calf Raises	8	50-100		
4. Ball Crunches	12	0-10		
Ball Crunches	10	0-10		
Ball Crunches	8	0-10		
5. Ball V-Ups	12	0		
Ball V-Ups	10	0		
Ball V-Ups	8	0		

Week 3 - Wednesday
Food Menu

Today's Menu	What I Ate
1. 2-3 Egg Omelet 100% Whole Wheat Toast	
2. Protein Shake	
3. Grilled Chicken Sandwich Piece of Fruit or Vegetables	
4. Protein Shake	
5. Grilled Fish Steamed Vegetables Brown Rice	
6. Protein Shake or Bar	

Week 3 - Wednesday
Cardio Activity
20-40 Minutes

Week 3 - Thursday
Food Menu

Today's Menu	What I Ate
1. 2-3 Eggs 1-2 Pancakes	
2. Protein Shake	

3. Chili
    Whole Wheat Crackers
    Side Salad	

4. Protein Shake	

5. Pork Chops or Chicken
    Steamed Vegetables
    Baked Potato	

6. Protein Shake or Bar	

74

Week 3: Pyramid-up
Workout 3
-Back, Biceps -

Exercise	Your Goal		Your Set	
	Reps x Weight		Reps x Weight	
1. Lat Pulldowns*	12	30-60		
Lat Pulldowns	10	30-60		
Lat Pulldowns	8	30-60		
2. Pullovers	12	8-15		
Pullovers	10	8-15		
Pullovers	8	8-15		
3. 2 DB Rows	12	8-15		
2 DB Rows	10	8-15		
2 DB Rows	8	8-15		
4. Hammer Curls	12	8-15		
Hammer Curls	10	8-15		
Hammer Curls	8	8-15		
5. BB Curls	12	15-30		
BB Curls	10	15-30		
BB Curls	8	15-30		

*Wide Grip

Week 3 - Friday
Food Menu

Today's Menu	What I Ate
1. Protein Shake	
2. Plain Yogurt Grape Nuts Banana	
3. Turkey Wrap	
4. Protein Shake	
5. Broiled Seafood Side Salad Sourdough Bread	
6. Protein Shake or Bar	

Week 3: Pyramid-up
Workout 4
-Abs, Arms -

Exercise	Your Goal		Your Set	
	Reps x	Weight	Reps x	Weight
1. Rev Crunch	F	0		
Rev Crunch	F	0		
Rev Crunch	F	0		
2. SkullKrushers	12	5-15		
SkullKrushers	10	5-15		
SkullKrushers	8	5-15		
3. DB Curls	12	8-15		
DB Curls	10	8-15		
DB Curls	8	8-15		
4. Tricep Ext.	12	10-20		
Tricep Ext.	10	10-20		
Tricep Ext.	8	10-20		
5. Ab Bench Crunch	12	0		
Ab Bench Crunch	10	0		
Ab Bench Crunch	8	0		

Week 3 - Saturday
Food Menu

Today's Menu	What I Ate
1. Protein Shake	

2. Baked Potato
    Cottage Cheese
    Turkey Breast	

3. Tunafish Sandwich	
4. Protein Shake	
5. Grilled Chicken Salad	
6. Protein Shake or Bar	

Week 3 - Saturday
No Organized Exercise

Week 3 - Sunday
Food Menu

Today's Menu	What I Ate
1. Hard Boiled Eggs Fruit	
2. Protein Shake	
3. Pizza or Pasta!!!	
4. Protein Shake	
5. Stir-fry	
6. Nothing!	

Week 3 - Sunday
Cardio Activity
20-45 Minutes

Sometimes telling people that you are starting a new fitness program can give you a little extra support & motivation.

Week 4: Fat Melting Week

Are you ready to have some real fun!

After 3 weeks of a solid weight training foundation you should be comfortable with lifting weights and seeing some nice results. Especially you should notice an increase in strength and firmness.

Now it is time to melt away a layer of fat!

One of the best ways to LOSE FAT AND GAIN MUSCLE is to follow a proven weight training program, eat right most of the time and occasionally, do a 5-day low carb week.

Please note: Doing low carbs all the time has some very negative consequences, one of the main ones is that you will gain all the weight back you lost PLUS more as soon as you start eating normal again! And with few exceptions, everybody goes back to eating normal.

A hidden secret is to eat low carbs for only 5 days, done at the right time and combine it with a weight training program. This will do wonders for your body. It is the one way to lose fat and gain muscle fast. It has a drug like effect, with absolutely no drugs.

It is simple to perform. But not easy mentally or physically. The nice thing is it is only 5 days of eating no or low carbohydrates. Most people can handle 5 days.

Done correctly, you can lose 2-4 pounds of fat in 5 days. Plus you will add new lean muscle the following week. What's better than that?!

Here is how to do it.

Starting late Sunday, do not eat any food with carbohydrates in them. Weight train hard on Monday. Do cardiovascular activity on Tuesday, Wednesday and Thursday. Weight train later in the day Friday. Then start eating normal again.

THAT'S IT!

Week 4: Fat Melting Week

Pretty simple. But you will get hungry, especially the first couple of days. After you become used to no carbs, then your hunger will subside.

Briefly, this is what happens. (If you want more detailed info on low carb diets, check out *The Atkins Diet, Protein Power* or *BodyOpus* books.)

Your body normally runs on carbs(sugar or blood sugar, ie. glucose}. When your carbs get low, your body needs a new fuel source to run on. It will then start using ketones. Ketones are a fuel made from fat. Your body breaks down fat into ketones, to use as fuel. This is called ketosis and it is very inefficient way to power your body. This is good news for you. It takes a lot of fat to make those ketones. Which means a lot of fat loss for you!!

When you are in ketosis, the body also tries to conserve muscle from being lost. Another big bonus that a regular calorie cutting diets do not do.

Last, but not least, when you start eating carbs again and following the weight training program, your muscles are like a huge sponge and super-compensation occurs. You will add new lean muscle. You will break through old plateaus. Your muscles will pull in more carbs and protein than normal. YOUR BODY WILL CHANGE!

Low Carb Foods

I am going to give you a food menu of close to zero carbohydrates. There are a few choices but it is a fairly small menu. The grocery store has some packaged low carb foods that could be another option. Use whatever works for you. It is only 5 days!

The key is to consume less than 20-30 grams of carbs a day. The lower the better. Make sure to check food labels for hidden cabs. If you are not hungry, do not eat. Drink water instead.

Week 4: Fat Melting Week

Menu

<u>MEAT</u>
Chicken
Turkey
Beef
Pork
Fish
Seafood
- Watch for processed meats, many could have added sugar.

<u>EGGS</u>
Or Egg substitute

<u>DAIRY</u>
Hard Cheeses - Has a few carbs so do not consume over 5 ounces.
Cream
Half/Half
Sour Cream

<u>BUTTER, OILS, SALAD DRESSING</u>

<u>VEGETABLES</u>
Lettuce/Spinach/Sprouts
Celery
Cucumber
Radishes
Peppers
Mushrooms
Avocado

<u>SNACKS</u>
Fried Pork Rinds, Sugar Free Jell-O, Sugar Free Gum, Jerky

<u>BEVERAGES</u>
Water, Tea, Coffee, Diet Sodas & Drinks

Week 4: Fat Melting Week

IMPORTANT

*If you do not feel comfortable doing the low carb diet or want to skip it this week, this is not a problem. It is the fastest way to lose fat but is not necessary for success with this program.

*If you need to quit low carbs before finishing the full 5 days, do it. Sometimes your body or schedule is not up to doing low carbs. Just go back to the normal food menu.

*Do not do the low carb diet more than one week per month. Doing it too often is hard on your body, hard to add lean muscle and loses its effectiveness.

*If you have any health issues, please consult with your doctor before starting any new diet plan.

Week 4

- Two workouts. One HARD workout Monday.
- Second workout on Friday.
- Pyramid-up workouts again.
- 5 exercises per workout.
- 3 sets per exercise.
- 12-10-8 reps.
- Rest 2-3 minutes between sets. When you rest up to three minutes between sets, you reclaim most of your strength. This allows you to perform the maximum amount of reps on your next set.
- Cardio hard three days!
- Go to muscle fatigue on the weight training workouts!

Find low/no carbohydrate snacks. There are several in the grocery store and many on the internet that will help you through the 5 days of losing fat!

Week 4 – Monday
Food Menu

Today's Menu	What I Ate
1. 2-3 eggs	
2. Ham String Cheese	
3. Hot Dog Pickles	
4. Skip Meal Diet Soda/Water	
5. Grilled Fish Lettuce/Cheese Salad	
6. Pumpkin Seeds	

Week 4: Pyramid-up
Workout 1
-Total Body-

Exercise	Your Goal		Your Set	
	Reps x	Weight	Reps x	Weight
1. Leg Press	12	50-100		
Leg Press	10	50-100		
Leg Press	8	50-100		
2. Pullovers	12	10-20		
Pullovers	10	10-20		
Pullovers	8	10-20		
3. Bench Press	12	25-45		
Bench Press	10	25-45		
Bench Press	8	25-45		
4. Lat Pulldown*	12	10-20		
Lat Pulldown	10	10-20		
Lat Pulldown	8	10-20		
5. BB Squats	12	30-60		
BB Squats	10	30-60		
BB Squats	8	30-60		

*Triangle Bar

Week 4 – Tuesday
Food Menu

Today's Menu	What I Ate
1. Coffee/Tea/Water	
2. Bacon String Cheese	
3. Skip Meal Diet Soda/Water	
4. Steak Lettuce/Cheese Salad	
5. Fried Pork Rinds	
6. Skip Meal	

Week 4 – Tuesday
Cardio Activity
20-45 Minutes

Week 4 - Wednesday
Food Menu

Today's Menu	What I Ate
1. 2 Hard Boiled Eggs	
2. Celery W/Peanut Butter	
3. Chicken Breast	
4. Sugar Free Jell-O	
5. Cocktail Shrimp	
6. Diet Soda/Tea	

Week 4 – Wednesday
Cardio Activity
20-45 Minutes

Week 4 – Thursday
Food Menu

Today's Menu	What I Ate
1. Omelet Made W/Half&Half	
2. Diet/Coffee/Water	
3. No Bun Cheeseburger Pickels	
4. Cottage Cheese	
5. Grilled Tuna or Canned Tuna with Mayo & Pickles	
6. Diet Soda/Tea	

Thursday
Cardio Activity
20-45 Minutes

Week 4 – Friday
Food Menu

Today's Menu	What I Ate
1. Ham & Eggs	
2. Fried Pork Rinds	
3. Grilled Chicken Salad	
4. Cheese Olives	
5. *AFTER YOUR WORKOUT* Protein Shake W/Carbs	
6. Whatever You Want- Pig Out!!!!	

Week 4: Pyramid-up
Workout 2
-Total Body-

Exercise	Your Goal		Your Set	
	Reps x Weight		Reps x Weight	
. Walking Lunges	F	5-20		
Walking Lunges	F	5-20		
Walking Lunges	F	5-20		
. Lat Pulldowns*	12	30-50		
Lat Pulldowns	10	30-50		
Lat Pulldowns	8	30-50		
. Tri. Pushdowns	12	15-30		
Tri. Pushdowns	10	15-30		
Tri. Pushdowns	8	15-30		
. BB Curl	12	15-30		
BB Curl	10	15-30		
BB Curl	8	15-30		
. BB Press	12	15-30		
BB Press	10	15-30		
BB Press	8	15-30		

Underhand Grip

Week 4 – Saturday
Food Menu

Today's Menu	What I Ate
1. Bowl of Cereal	
2. Protein Shake	
3. Pizza	
4. Protein Shake	
5. Pasta Meal	
6. Glass of Wine or Beer or Juice	

Week 4 – Saturday
Relax and Have Fun!

Week 4 - Sunday
Food Menu

Today's Menu	What I Ate
Meal 1: Protein Shake	
Meal 2: Baked Potato **Cottage Cheese** **Turkey Breast**	
Meal 3: Protein Shake	
Meal 4: Peanut Butter Sandwich **Whole Wheat Bread**	
Meal 5: Baked Fish **Steamed Vegetables**	
Meal 6: Protein Shake	

Week 4 – Sunday
No Organized Activity

The best medicine is not in a bottle-it's in proper exercise, a wholesome diet and in your head!

How did the low carb week go?

Not easy is it….but I bet you lost a lot of weight and kept off a few pounds!

You should have lost about 5-10 pounds. Two-thirds will be water weight that comes back when you start eating carbs again. BUT 2-4 lbs will be fat. In 5 days that is unbeatable! Plus you saved your hard-earned muscle and will be adding more this week.

Now your body is ready to add lean muscle like you have never seen before. It will use the quality food you are eating and pump it into your starving muscles. Return to eating good, quality food along with your 2-3 protein shakes a day. Eat more this week. This is the week you want to add fat burning muscle.

Remember-
More carbs the 1st half of the day….less carbs the 2nd half.
More carbs before and after weight training.
Less carbs before and after cardio activity.

Your muscles are rested, hungry and ready to grow, so you are going to weight train 5x this week using Super Sets.

Super Sets are probably the most performed workout routine ever. They are arguably the best all-time way to weight train and for a very good reason. They work and they are simple. Super Sets allow you attack specific muscles and force them to grow. This works fantastic for the average person who has a hard time taking straight sets to muscle failure, which most people do.

Week 5: Super Sets

Super Sets are 2 different exercises done in a row with no rest in between. The best way to use Super Sets is to target the same muscles or opposing muscle groups.

Example: Same muscle group.

BB Bench Press
to (no rest)
Incline DB Bench Press

This would be a chest to chest workout.

Example: Opposing muscle group.

Tricep Pushdowns
to (no rest)
BB Curls

This would be a tricep to bicep workout.

The two exercises should be as close together as possible in proximity, so you can do them back to back with no rest.

Week 5

- Five workouts. Your body is primed to add muscle!
- 6 or 7 Super Sets per workout.
- 8-12 reps per set.
- Rest 2-4 minutes between Super Sets.
- No rest during Super Set.
- Go to muscle failure.
- Use a spotter if available!

Week 5 - Monday
Food Menu

Today's Menu	What I Ate
1. 2-3 Eggs 2 100% Whole Wheat Toast	
2. Baked Potato Cottage Cheese Turkey Breast	
3. Protein Shake	
4. Handful of Nuts Piece of Fruit	
5. Baked Fish Steamed Vegetables Brown Rice	
6. Protein Shake	

Week 5: Super Sets
Workout 1
-Chest-

Exercise	Your Goal		Your Set	
	Reps x Weight		Reps x Weight	
1. Incline Flys	8	8-15		
DB Press	8	10-20		
2. Incline Flys	8	8-15		
DB Press	8	10-20		
3. Incline Flys	8	8-15		
DB Press	8	10-20		
. Incline DB Bench	8	8-20		
BB Bench Press	8	30-50		
. Incline DB Bench	8	8-20		
BB Bench Press	8	30-50		
. Incline DB Bench	8	8-20		
BB Bench Press	8	30-50		
. Incline DB Press	8	15-30*		
. Incline DB Press	8	15-30*		

ingles sets. Heavy weights. Rest 3 minutes between sets.
it muscle fatigue on or before the 8th rep.

Week 5 - Tuesday
Food Menu

Today's Menu	What I Ate
1. Plain Yogurt with Grapenuts and Fruit	
2. Turkey Sandwich on 100% Whole Wheat Bread Baked Chips	
3. Protein Shake	
4. Celery with Peanut Butter	
5. Grilled Chicken Salad Light Dressing	
6. Protein Bar or Glass of Milk	

Week 5: Super Sets
Workout 2
-Legs-

Exercise	Your Goal		Your Set	
	Reps x Weight		Reps x Weight	
1. Leg Curl	10	25-50		
Walking Lunges	F	5-20		
2. Leg Curl	10	25-50		
Walking Lunges	F	5-20		
3. Leg Curl	10	25-50		
Walking Lunges	F	5-20		
4. Leg Ext.	15	25-50		
BB Squats	10	30-50		
5. Leg Ext.	15	25-50		
BB Squats	10	30-50		
6. Calf Raises*	15	50-100		
Leg Press	8	50-100		
7. Calf Raises*	15	50-100		
Leg Press	8	50-100		

Do Calf Raises on the Leg Press Machine.

Week 5 - Wednesday
Food Menu

Today's Menu	What I Ate
1. 2-3 Eggs Baked Potato	
2. Turkey Jerky	
3. Tuna Fish Sandwich on Whole Wheat Bread	
4. Protein Shake	
5. Lean Hamburger Steamed Vegetables	
6. Glass of Milk or Yogurt	

Week 5: Super Sets
Workout 3
-Abs-

Exercise	Your Goal Reps x Weight		Your Set Reps x Weight	
1. Rev Crunch	F	0		
Ball Crunch	15	0		
2. Rev Crunch	F	0		
Ball Crunch	15	0		
3. Rev Crunch	F	0		
Ball Crunch	15	0		
4. Ab Bench Crunch	10	0		
Ball V-Ups	10	0		
5. Ab Bench Crunch	10	0		
Ball V-Ups	10	0		
6. Ab Bench Crunch	10	0		
Ball V-Ups	10	0		

Week 5 - Thursday
Food Menu

Today's Menu	What I Ate
1. Protein Shake	
2. String Cheese Raw Vegetables	
3. Turkey Wrap	
4. Cup of Cottage Cheese Piece of Fruit	
5. Bowl of Chili Whole Wheat Crackers	
6. Protein Bar or Handful of Deli Turkey/Roast Beef	

Week 5 - Thursday
Light Cardio
15-30 Minutes

Week 5 - Friday
Food Menu

Today's Menu	What I Ate
1. Oatmeal with Raisins	
2. Protein Shake	
3. Grilled Chicken Breast Coleslaw	
4. Cottage Cheese Bowl of Fruit	
5. Grilled Steak Salad	
6. Protein Shake	

Week 5: Super Sets
Workout 4
-Back-

Exercise	Your Goal Reps x Weight		Your Set Reps x Weight	
1. Pullovers	8	15-30		
Lat Pulldown*	8	40-80		
2. Pullovers	8	15-30		
Lat Pulldown*	8	40-80		
3. Pullovers	8	15-30		
Lat Pulldown*	8	40-80		
4. Pullovers	8	15-30		
Lat Pulldown*	8	40-80		
5. Deadlifts	10	10-45		
2 DB Rows	10	10-20		
6. Deadlifts	10	10-45		
2 DB Rows	10	10-20		

Wide Grip

Week 5 - Saturday
Food Menu

Today's Menu	What I Ate
1. 2-3 eggs Whole Grain English Muffin	
2. Protein Shake	
3. Bowl of Soup Side Salad 1 Whole Wheat Bread	
4. Apple & Cheese	
5. Broiled Shrimp Steamed Vegetables	
6. Protein Bar	

Week 5: Super Sets
Workout 5
-Triceps-

Exercise	Your Goal		Your Set	
	Reps x	Weight	Reps x	Weight
1. SkullKrushers	12	8-15		
Kickbacks	12	5-10		
2. SkullKrushers	12	8-15		
Kickbacks	12	5-10		
3. SkullKrushers	12	8-15		
Kickbacks	12	5-10		
4. Tricep Ext.	12	8-15		
Pushdowns	12	15-30		
5. Tricep Ext.	12	8-15		
Pushdowns	12	15-30		
6. Tricep Ext.	12	8-15		
Pushdowns	12	15-30		

Week 5 - Sunday
Food Menu

Today's Menu	What I Ate
1. Waffle & Sugar Free Syrup Turkey Ham	
2. Baked Potato Roast Beef Cottage Cheese	
3. Grilled Chicken Salad	
4. Fruit & Yogurt	
5. Tuna Fish Sandwich on Whole Wheat Bread Raw Vegetables	
6. Protein Shake	

118

Week 5 - Sunday
Rest Day!

Learn to cook and like it!

Week 6: Super Sets

You should be seeing major changes in your physical appearance. Clothes fitting better, new muscles you never knew existed, muscle definition and a tightness around your body that feels incredible!

You will also notice an increase in your appetite. A deep physical hunger in your stomach that needs to be fed. <u>This is a good thing</u>. Your metabolism is cranking up from the 6 small meals a day and proven workouts. You are burning more calories, building new muscle and turning your body into a fat burning machine.

Keep it up! Just make sure you are following the food plan as close to possible for maximum results.

Eat a little less than you did in Week 5 to keep that fat melting.

You will continue with Super Sets in Week 6 with four workouts.

You are going to be much stronger now and need to try and take each set to muscle fatigue. TRY 3 MORE REPS WHEN YOU DO NOT WANT TO DO ANYMORE! This is when your body will change. These changes happen fast because your body has to be able to perform the exercise better next time you ask it to do it. It is that simple to building more fat free muscle.

Remember to warm up, take every set to muscle fatigue and keep breathing properly!

Week 6: Super Sets

Week 6

- Three workouts.
- Non-consecutive days.
- 6 Super Sets per workout.
- No rest during Super Set
- 8-12 reps per set.
- Try to have the 2 exercises close together.
- Warm up! Breathe! Slow negatives!

Prepare your meals ahead of time so you can eat healthy while away from home. Invest in plastic containers.

Week 6 - Monday
Food Menu

Today's Menu	What I Ate
1. 2-3 eggs 100% Whole Wheat Toast	
2. Protein Shake	
3. Grilled Chicken Salad	
4. Protein Shake	
5. Baked Fish Brown Rice Steamed Vegetables	
6. String Cheese	

Week 6: Super Sets
Workout 1
-Biceps-

Exercise	Your Goal Reps x Weight		Your Set Reps x Weight	
1. BB Curls	12	15-30		
Cable Curls*	12	15-30		
2. BB Curls	12	15-30		
Cable Curls*	12	15-30		
3. BB Curls	12	15-30		
Cable Curls*	12	15-30		
4. Hammer Curls	12	8-15		
Cable Curls**	12	15-30		
5. Hammer Curls	12	8-15		
Cable Curls**	12	15-30		
6. Hammer Curls	12	8-15		
Cable Curls**	12	15-30		

Use the Bar Attachment
Use the Rope Attachment

Week 6 - Tuesday
Food Menu

Today's Menu	What I Ate
1. Protein Shake	
2. Baked Potato Cottage Cheese Black Olives	
3. Turkey Sandwich Banana	
4. Protein Shake	
5. Grilled Lean Steak Side Salad	
6. Glass of Milk or Yogurt	

Week 6 - Tuesday
Cardio Activity
20-45 Minutes

Week 6 - Wednesday
Food Menu

Today's Menu	What I Ate
1. Protein Shake	
2. Cottage Cheese Bowl of Fruit	
3. Lean Hamburger Baked Chips	
4. Protein Shake	
5. Grilled Chicken Breast Sweet Potato/Yam	
6. Glass of Milk or Yogurt or Nuts	

Week 6: Super Sets
Workout 2
-Legs-

Exercise	Your Goal Reps x Weight		Your Set Reps x Weight	
1. Leg Press	15	50-100		
Leg Ext.	15	25-40		
2. Leg Press	15	50-100		
Leg Ext.	15	25-40		
3. Deadlifts	10	10-45		
Walking Lunges	F	5-20		
4. Deadlifts	10	10-45		
Walking Lunges	F	5-20		
5. Leg Curl	10	25-50		
Leg Ext.	15	25-40		
6. Leg Curl	10	25-50		
Leg Ext.	15	25-40		

F: Muscle fatigue. You can NOT do any more reps with good form.

Week 6 - Thursday
Food Menu

Today's Menu	What I Ate
1. Oatmeal with Milk	
2. Celery w/Peanut Butter	
3. Protein Shake	
4. String Cheese	
5. Fajitas	
6. Protein Shake	

Week 6 - Thursday
Cardio Activity
20-45 Minutes

Week 6 - Friday
Food Menu

Today's Menu	What I Ate
1. Omelet Whole Wheat Toast	
2. Protein Shake	
3. Tuna Fish Sandwich Raw Vegetables	
4. Protein Shake	
5. Grilled Chicken Brown Rice Side Salad	
6. Glass of Milk or Yogurt	

Week 6: Super Sets
Workout 3
-Shoulders-

Exercise	Your Goal Reps x Weight		Your Set Reps x Weight	
1. Rear Raise	10	3-10		
DB Press	10	8-15		
2. Rear Raise	10	3-10		
DB Press	10	8-15		
3. Front Raise	10	3-10		
BB Press	10	15-30		
4. Front Raise	10	3-10		
BB Press	10	15-30		
5. Side Raise	8	3-10		
BB Press	8	15-30		
6. Side Raise	8	3-10		
BB Press	8	15-30		

Week 6 - Saturday
Food Menu

Today's Menu	What I Ate
1. Protein Shake	
2. Piece of Fruit & Nuts	
3. Grilled Chicken Sandwich Baked Beans	
4. Protein Shake	
5. Grilled Fish Steamed Vegetables Baked Yam	
6. Jerky	

Week 6 - Saturday
Cardio Activity
20-45 Minutes

Week 6 - Sunday
Food Menu

Today's Menu	What I Ate
1. Roast Beef Baked potato Melted Cheese	
2. Protein Shake	
3. Turkey Sandwich	
4. Protein Shake	
5. Grilled Chicken Brown Rice Side Salad	
6. Yogurt or Protein Bar	

Week 6 - Sunday
Rest!

Week 7: 3-in-a-Row

Seven weeks into building your new body, this program should start to be a habit. Habits take 1-2 months to establish. That is the hard part. Then it is just what you do. What you are. Who you are. That is where you should be now!

Continue eating 6 small meals a day, mostly natural foods, protein shakes, plus a little cardio and your weight training workouts should feel like home now! Additionally you are not hungry, very healthy and your lifestyle is still intact.

You are going to lift hard one more week and next week you will be able to back off on the weight training.

Ready to feel your muscles explode? 3-in-a-Row will do the trick! This workout has been refined from years of research, practice and teaching. Here is what I discovered: IT WORKS. No complicated math, calculators or stop watches. Just results!

<u>3-in-a-Row</u>

- Same exercise.
- Same weight.
- Same rep goal.
- 3 sets.
- 30 seconds rest between the 3 sets.
- Rest up to 5 minutes before start the next 3-in-a-Row.

Example

Set 1. Incline DB Curls – 10 Reps x 20 lbs.
    Rest only 30 seconds.
    Incline DB Curls – 10 Reps x 20 lbs.
    Rest only 30 seconds.
    Incline DB Curls – 10 Reps x 20 lbs.
    Rest 3-5 minutes. Start next 3-in-a-Row.

You will probably be unable to reach you rep goal on the 2nd and 3rd set. GOOD! This is suppose to happen and it tells your body you do not have enough muscle and strength to finish the sets. This will turn on your muscle building machine. You will get fit & firm fast.

Keep eating your six small meals every day. Shoot for about 1 gram of protein per pound of body weight per day. If you are following the food menus, you will be getting ample amounts of protein.

Week 7

- Three workouts
- 5 exercises per workout.
- 8-15 reps per set.
- Rest 30 seconds during 3-in-a-Row.
- Rest up to 5 minutes between sets.
- Use a spotter if available.
- Use perfect form.
- Warm up! Breathe! Slow negatives!

Week 7 - Monday
Food Menu

Today's Menu	What I Ate
1. Protein Shake	
2. Celery with Peanut Butter	
3. Grilled Chicken Sandwich	
4. Protein Shake	
5. Turkey Wrap	
6. Protein Shake or Bar	

Week 7: 3-in-a-Row
Workout 1
-Back & Biceps-

Exercise	Your Goal		Your Set	
	Reps x	Weight	Reps x	Weight
1. 2 DB Pullovers	10	8-15		
2 DB Pullovers	10	8-15		
2 DB Pullovers	10	8-15		
2. 2 DB Pullovers	10	8-15		
2 DB Pullovers	10	8-15		
2 DB Pullovers	10	8-15		
3. Lat Pulldown*	10	30-60		
Lat Pulldown	10	30-60		
Lat Pulldown	10	30-60		
4. DB Curls	15	8-20		
DB Curls	15	8-20		
DB Curls	15	8-20		
5. Incline Curls	10	8-15		
Incline Curls	10	8-15		
Incline Curls	10	8-15		

*Triangle Bar

Week 7 - Tuesday
Food Menu

Today's Menu	What I Ate
1. Protein Shake	
2. Baked Potato Cottage Cheese Turkey Breast	
3. Yogurt with Fruit	
4. Protein Shake	
5. Lean Steak or Chicken Steamed Vegetables 2 Whole Wheat Bread	
6. Protein Shake or Bar	

Week 7 - Tuesday
Cardio Activity
20-40 Minutes

Week 7 - Wednesday
Food Menu

Today's Menu	What I Ate
1. 2-3 Egg Omelet 100% Whole Wheat Toast	
2. Protein Shake	
3. Grilled Chicken Sandwich Piece of Fruit or Vegetables	
4. Protein Shake	
5. Grilled Fish Steamed Vegetables Brown Rice	
6. Protein Shake or Bar	

Week 7: 3-in-a-Row
Workout 2
-Legs, Abs-

Exercise	Your Goal		Your Set	
	Reps x	Weight	Reps x	Weight
. Leg Ext.	15	30-50		
Leg Ext.	15	30-50		
Leg Ext.	15	30-50		
. BB Squats	10	30-60		
BB Squats	10	30-60		
BB Squats	10	30-60		
. BB Squats	10	30-60		
BB Squats	10	30-60		
BB Squats	10	30-60		
. Leg Press	15	60-120		
Leg Press	15	60-120		
Leg Press	15	60-120		
. Crunches	15	0		
Crunches	15	0		
Crunches	15	0		

Week 7 - Thursday
Food Menu

Today's Menu	What I Ate
1. 2-3 Eggs 1-2 Pancakes	
2. Protein Shake	

3. Chili
   Whole Wheat Crackers
   Side Salad	

4. Protein Shake	

5. Pork Chops
   Steamed Vegetables
   Baked Potato	

6. Protein Shake or Bar	

Week 7 - Thursday
Cardio Activity
20-40 Minutes

\

Week 7 - Friday
Food Menu

Today's Menu	What I Ate
1. Protein Shake	
2. Plain Yogurt Grape Nuts Banana	
3. Turkey Wrap	
4. Protein Shake	
5. Broiled Seafood Side Salad Sourdough Bread	
6. Protein Shake or Bar	

148

Week 7: 3-in-a-Row
Workout 3
-Chest, Shoulders, Triceps-

Exercise	Your Goal		Your Set	
	Reps x Weight		Reps x Weight	
BB Bench Press	8	30-50		
BB Bench Press	8	30-50		
BB Bench Press	8	30-50		
BB Bench Press	8	30-50		
BB Bench Press	8	30-50		
BB Bench Press	8	30-50		
BB Press	10	20-40		
BB Press	10	20-40		
BB Press	10	20-40		
BB Press	10	20-40		
BB Press	10	20-40		
BB Press	10	20-40		
Pushdowns	10	20-40		
Pushdowns	10	20-40		
Pushdowns	10	20-40		

Week 7 - Saturday
Food Menu

Today's Menu	What I Ate
1. Protein Shake	
2. Baked Potato Cottage Cheese Turkey Breast	
3. Tunafish Sandwich	
4. Protein Shake	
5. Grilled Chicken Salad	
6. Protein Shake or Bar	

Week 7 - Saturday
Rest

Week 7 - Sunday
Food Menu

Today's Menu	What I Ate
1. Hard Boiled Eggs Fruit	
2. Protein Shake	
3. Pizza or Pasta!!!	
4. Protein Shake	
5. Stir-fry	
6. Nothing!	

Week 7 - Sunday
Rest

Find a workout partner!

Week 8: 3-in-a-Row

Time to melt away more fat and see your new muscles! Week 8 will be your 2nd round of low carbohydrates. This time you should feel more comfortable choosing low carb foods and sticking with the simple plan.

You will be lifting weights hard Monday to push your body into Ketosis and then doing only cardio the rest of the week. Your body needs a small break from weight training every 2 months, so you will not lift weights again until Week 9.

Remember to only eat when you are really hungry and drink lots of water. Do your cardio 4x and you should be able to LOSE 2-3 pounds of fat this week!!

Week 8

- 1 workout, <u>beginning of the week</u>.
- Continue 3-in-a-Row workouts.
- Total body workout.
- Go to failure on every set.
- *Cardio exercise for the remainder of the week.*
- Keep carbs under 20 grams per day!
- Start eating carbs again Friday PM.

Week 8 – Monday
Food Menu

Today's Menu	What I Ate
1. 2-3 eggs	
2. Ham String Cheese	
3. Hot Dog Pickles	
4. Skip Meal Diet Soda/Water	
5. Grilled Fish Lettuce/Cheese Salad	
6. Pumpkin Seeds	

Week 8: 3-in-a-Row
Workout 1
-Total Body-

Exercise	Your Goal Reps x Weight		Your Set Reps x Weight	
1. DB Curls	12	10-25		
DB Curls	12	10-25		
DB Curls	12	10-25		
2. Deadlifts	12	30-50		
Deadlifts	12	30-50		
Deadlifts	12	30-50		
3. 2 DB Rows	12	10-20		
2 DB Rows	12	10-20		
2 DB Rows	12	10-20		
4. Incline DB Bench	12	15-25		
Incline DB Bench	12	15-25		
Incline DB Bench	12	15-25		
5. DB Squats	15	15-30		
DB Squats	15	15-30		
DB Squats	15	15-30		

Week 8 – Tuesday
Food Menu

Today's Menu	What I Ate
1. Coffee/Tea/Water	
2. Bacon String Cheese	
3. Skip Meal Diet Soda/Water	
4. Steak Lettuce/Cheese Salad	
5. Fried Pork Rinds	
6. Skip Meal	

Week 8 - Tuesday
Cardio Activity
30-45 Minutes

Week 8 – Wednesday
Food Menu

Today's Menu	What I Ate
1. 2 Hard Boiled Eggs	
2. Celery w/Peanut Butter	
3. Chicken Breast	
4. Sugar Free Jell-O	
5. Cocktail Shrimp	
6. Diet Soda/Tea	

Week 8 - Wednesday
Cardio Activity
30-45 Minutes

Week 8 – Thursday
Food Menu

Today's Menu	What I Ate
1. Omelet Made w/Half&Half	
2. Diet/Coffee/Water	
3. No Bun Cheeseburger Pickels	
4. Cottage Cheese	
5. Grilled Tuna or Canned Tuna with Mayo & Pickles	
6. Diet Soda/Tea	

162

Week 8 - Thursday
Cardio Activity
30-45 Minutes

Week 8 – Friday
Food Menu

Today's Menu	What I Ate
1. Ham & Eggs	
2. Fried Pork Rinds	
3. Grilled Chicken Salad	
4. Cheese Black Olives	
5. *AFTER YOUR CARDIO* Protein Shake w/Carbs	
6. Whatever you want- Pig out!!!!	

Week 8 - Friday
Cardio Activity
30-45 Minutes

Week 8 – Saturday
Food Menu

Today's Menu	What I Ate
1. Bowl of Cereal	
2. Protein Shake	
3. Pizza	
4. Protein Shake	
5. Pasta Meal	
6. Glass of Wine or Beer and Nuts	

Week 8 - Saturday
REST!!

Week 8 – Sunday
Food Menu

Today's Menu	What I Ate
1. Protein Shake	
2. Cottage Cheese Bowl of Fruit	
3. Lean Hamburger Baked Chips	
4. Protein Shake	
5. Grilled Chicken Breast Sweet Potato/Yam	
6. Glass of Milk or Yogurt or Nuts	

168

Week 8 - Sunday
REST!!

Have a protein source with every meal.
If you don't, your body eats your hard
earned muscle for the protein!

Week 9: Drop Sets

Did you lose weight during the low carb week? 2, 3, 4 lbs? Are you seeing muscles and definition you never knew existed? You should be! If not, make sure you are only eating foods with no or very low carbs, watching out for condiments, processed food and beverages with hidden sugars.

AND DO YOUR CARDIO!

Week 9 - You are ready to add rock hard muscle like you have never seen. Your muscles are like a sponge from the low carb week, plus you took a week off from weight training. You are ready to bust through any plateau you might have hit.

You are going to weight train very hard this week plus eating a few more calories. Your body is primed for new progress. Don't waste this opportunity. This is what you have worked for...A NEW BODY!!!

Weeks 9 and 10 consist of Drop Sets. My personal all-time favorite muscle builder ever! If you do not add muscle, add strength and lose fat during the next two weeks, YOU DID NOT SHOW UP!

Drop Sets

- Perform exercise to muscle failure.
- With no rest, lower the weight ~30%.
- Perform same exercise to muscle failure.
- With no rest, lower the weight again ~30%.
- Perform same exercise to muscle failure.
- Rest up to 5 minutes before starting the next Drop Set.

Week 9: Drop Sets

Example: Leg Press

SET 1A): 100 lbs. X 12 reps
  ↓ no rest

SET 1B): 70 lbs. X 12 reps
  ↓ no rest

SET 1C): 50 lbs. X 12 reps
  Drop Set is complete
  Rest up to 5 minutes
  Go to the next Drop Set

Sound like fun!? Drop Sets can be taxing but really fatigue the muscle quickly and effectively for great gains. Drop Sets are most efficient if you have a workout partner to change the weights for you. If you do not have anyone around, just do the best you can.

Tip: The amount of weight you lower on each set will vary. Approximately a 30% drop on each set is the most effective. Each exercise and individual is different. You will have to experiment in the beginning to discover what works best for you.

Week 9: Drop Sets

Week 9

- Four workouts.
- 5 Drop Sets per workout.
- 5 exercises per workout.
- Rest 2-5 minutes after Drop Set.
- No rest during Drop Set!
- Take each set to fatigue.
- Eat good!

Week 9 - Monday
Food Menu

Today's Menu	What I Ate
1. 2-3 Eggs 2 100% Whole Wheat Toast	
2. Baked Potato Cottage Cheese Turkey Breast	
3. Protein Shake	
4. Handful of Nuts Piece of Fruit	
5. Baked Fish Steamed Vegetables Brown Rice	
6. Protein Shake	

Week 9: Drop Sets
Workout 1
-Arms-

Exercise	Your Goal		Your Set	
	Reps x	Weight	Reps x	Weight
1. SkullKrushers	10	12-20		
SkullKrushers	10	12-20		
SkullKrushers	10	12-20		
2. Incline Curls	10	10-15		
Incline Curls	10	10-15		
Incline Curls	10	10-15		
3. Pushdowns	10	20-40		
Pushdowns	10	20-40		
Pushdowns	10	20-40		
4. Cable Curls	10	20-40		
Cable Curls	10	20-40		
Cable Curls	10	20-40		
5. BB Curls	10	25-50		
BB Curls	10	25-50		
BB Curls	10	25-50		

Week 9 - Tuesday
Food Menu

Today's Menu	What I Ate
1. Protein Shake	
2. Baked Potato Cottage Cheese Black Olives	
3. Turkey Sandwich Banana	
4. Protein Shake	
5. Grilled Lean Steak Side Salad	
6. Glass of Milk or Yogurt	

Week 9: Drop Sets
Workout 2
-Legs-

Exercise	Your Goal		Your Set	
	Reps x Weight		Reps x Weight	
1. Leg Extensions	15	30-60		
Leg Extensions	15	30-60		
Leg Extensions	15	30-60		
2. Leg Extensions	15	30-60		
Leg Extensions	15	30-60		
Leg Extensions	15	30-60		
3. Leg Curls	10	30-60		
Leg Curls	10	30-60		
Leg Curls	10	30-60		
4. DB Squats	12	20-40		
DB Squats	12	20-40		
DB Squats	12	20-40		
5. DB Squats	8	20-40		
DB Squats	8	20-40		
DB Squats	8	20-40		

Week 9 - Wednesday
Food Menu

Today's Menu	What I Ate
1. 2-3 Eggs Baked Potato	
2. Turkey Jerky	
3. Tuna Fish Sandwich on 100% Whole Wheat Bread Baked Chips	
4. Protein Shake	
5. Lean Hamburger Steamed Vegetables	
6. Protein Shake	

Week 9 - Wednesday
No Cardio Today
Let Muscles Grow!

Week 9 - Thursday
Food Menu

Today's Menu	What I Ate
1. Protein Shake	
2. String Cheese Raw Vegetables	
3. Turkey Wrap	
4. Cup of Cottage Cheese Piece of Fruit	
5. Chicken Caesar Salad	
6. Protein Bar or Shake	

Week 9: Drop Sets
Workout 3
-Back, Chest-

Exercise	Your Goal Reps x Weight		Your Set Reps x Weight	
1. Rear Raise	10	8-15		
Rear Raise	10	8-15		
Rear Raise	10	8-15		
2. 2 DB Rows	10	15-30		
2 DB Rows	10	15-30		
2 DB Rows	10	30-60		
3. DB Bench Press	10	15-30		
DB Bench Press	10	15-30		
DB Bench Press	10	15-30		
4. 2 DB Rows	10	15-30		
2 DB Rows	10	15-30		
2 DB Rows	10	15-30		
5. BB Bench Press	8	45-70		
BB Bench Press	8	45-70		
BB Bench Press	8	45-70		

Week 9 - Friday
Food Menu

Today's Menu	What I Ate
1. Oatmeal with Raisins	
2. Protein Shake	
3. Grilled Chicken Breast Coleslaw	
4. Protein Shake or Bar	
5. Grilled Steak Salad	
6. Handful of Nuts	

Week 9: Drop Sets
Workout 4
-Legs & Shoulders-

Exercise	Your Goal Reps x Weight		Your Set Reps x Weight	
1. Calf Raise	15	75-125		
Calf Raise	15	75-125		
Calf Raise	15	75-125		
2. Leg Press	15	75-125		
Leg Press	15	75-125		
Leg Press	15	75-125		
3. Leg Press	15	75-125		
Leg Press	15	75-125		
Leg Press	15	75-125		
4. Side Raise	10	8-15		
Side Raise	10	8-15		
Side Raise	10	8-15		
5. BB Press	8	25-40		
BB Press	8	25-40		
BB Press	8	25-40		

Week 9 - Saturday
Food Menu

Today's Menu	What I Ate
1. 2-3 eggs Whole Grain English Muffin	
2. Protein Shake	

3. Bowl of Soup
   Side Salad
   1 Whole Wheat Bread	

4. Protein Shake	
5. Broiled Shrimp Steamed Vegetables	
6. Fruit or Nuts	

Week 9 - Saturday
Rest

Week 9 - Sunday
Food Menu

Today's Menu	What I Ate
1. Waffle & Sugar Free Syrup Turkey Ham	
2. Baked Potato Roast Beef Cottage Cheese	
3. Grilled Chicken Salad	
4. Fruit & Yogurt	
5. Tuna Fish Sandwich on Whole Wheat Bread Raw Vegetables	
6. Protein Shake	

Week 9 – Sunday
Cardio Activity
20-40 Minutes

Having a cheat meal occasionally is necessary. Having a cheat day is hard to recover from – make the smart choice!

Week 10: Drop Sets

Week 10 already! How do you look? Fabulous!

You should feel like a new person. Stronger, firmer, healthier and more confident in everything you do.

Just keep persistently following with the program. Results really go in spurts. You might not see much happening for a couple of weeks and all of sudden, BAM - you lose an inch on your waist and can fit into your favorite jeans again. Nothing better!

Make sure to keep eating your protein shakes. They are an important part of your menu. Try different brands if you are becoming tired of the same taste or consistency. Protein powders vary widely. Some are delicious. Some are not. It just depends on your taste.

Drop Sets one more week. Hopefully you were sore after your workouts last week? Remember - they work!

Week 10

- Three workouts.
- 5 Drop Sets per workout.
- 5 exercises per workout.
- Rest up to 5 minutes after Drop Set.
- No rest during Drop Set!
- 1 straight heavy set at the end of the workouts.
- Take each set to fatigue.
- Drink your protein shakes.

Week 10 - Monday
Food Menu

Today's Menu	What I Ate
1. 2-3 eggs 100% Whole Wheat Toast	
2. Protein Shake	
3. Grilled Chicken Salad	
4. Protein Shake	
5. Baked Fish Brown Rice Steamed Vegetables	
6. String Cheese	

Week 10: Drop Sets
Workout 1
-Abs, Back, Biceps-

Exercise	Your Goal Reps x Weight		Your Set Reps x Weight	
1. Ab Bench Crunch	15	0-25		
Ab Bench Crunch	15	0-25		
Ab Bench Crunch	15	0-25		
2. 2 DB Pullovers	10	8-15		
2 DB Pullovers	10	8-15		
2 DB Pullovers	10	8-15		
3. DB Pullovers	10	15-30		
DB Pullovers	10	15-30		
DB Pullovers	10	15-30		
4. BB Curls	10	20-30		
BB Curls	10	20-30		
BB Curls	10	20-30		
5. Incline Curls	8	8-15		
Incline Curls	8	8-15		
Incline Curls	8	8-15		
6. Lat Pullldown*	8	Heavy		

Triangle Bar. 1 heavy set. Muscle fatigue on or before the 8th rep.

Week 10 - Tuesday
Food Menu

Today's Menu	What I Ate
1. Protein Shake	
2. Baked Potato Cottage Cheese Black Olives	
3. Turkey Sandwich Banana	
4. Protein Shake	
5. Grilled Lean Steak Side Salad	
6. Glass of Milk or Yogurt	

Week 10 – Tuesday
Cardio Activity
20-40 Minutes

Week 10 - Wednesday
Food Menu

Today's Menu	What I Ate
1. Protein Shake	
2. Cottage Cheese Bowl of Fruit	
3. Lean Hamburger Baked Chips	
4. Protein Shake	

5. Grilled Chicken Breast
   Sweet Potato/Yam
   Side Salad	

6. Glass of Milk or Yogurt or Nuts	

Week 10: Drop Sets
Workout 2
-Abs, Legs-

Exercise	Your Goal Reps x Weight		Your Set Reps x Weight	
1. Ball V-Ups	15	0-25		
Ball V-Ups	15	0-25		
Ball V-Ups	15	0-25		
2. Leg Curls	8	40-70		
Leg Curls	8	40-70		
Leg Curls	8	40-70		
3. Leg Curls	8	40-70		
Leg Curls	8	40-70		
Leg Curls	8	40-70		
4. Leg Curls	8	40-70		
Leg Curls	8	40-70		
Leg Curls	8	40-70		
5. Walking Lunges	F	10-25		
Walking Lunges	F	10-25		
Walking Lunges	F	10-25		
6. BB Squats	15	45-70*		

set. Muscle fatigue on or before the 15th rep.

Week 10 - Thursday
Food Menu

Today's Menu	What I Ate
1. Oatmeal with Milk	
2. Celery w/ Peanut Butter	
3. Protein Shake	
4. String Cheese	
5. Fajitas	
6. Protein Shake	

Week 10 – Thursday
Cardio Activity
20-40 Minutes

Week 10 - Friday
Food Menu

Today's Menu	What I Ate
1. Omelet Whole Wheat Toast	
2. Protein Shake	
3. Tuna Fish Sandwich Raw Vegetables	
4. Protein Shake	

5. Grilled Chicken
   Brown Rice
   Side Salad	

6. Glass of Milk or Yogurt	

Week 10: Drop Sets
Workout 3
-Abs, Chest, Shoulders, Triceps-

Exercise	Your Goal		Your Set	
	Reps x Weight		Reps x Weight	
. Ball Crunches	15	0-25		
Ball Crunches	15	0-25		
Ball Crunches	15	0-25		
. DB Press	8	10-20		
DB Press	8	10-20		
DB Press	8	10-20		
. Side Raise	8	5-15		
Side Raise	8	5-15		
Side Raise	8	5-15		
. Incline DB Bench	8	12-20		
Incline DB Bench	8	12-20		
Incline DB Bench	8	12-20		
. Pushdowns	12	20-40		
Pushdowns	12	20-40		
Pushdowns	12	20-40		
. BB Bench	8	45-70*		

set. Muscle fatigue on or before the 8th rep.

Week 10 - Saturday
Food Menu

Today's Menu	What I Ate
1. Protein Shake	
2. Piece of Fruit & Nuts	
3. Grilled Chicken Sandwich Baked Beans	
4. Protein Shake	

5. Grilled Fish
   Steamed Vegetables
   Baked Yam	

6. Jerky	

Week 10 – Saturday
Rest!

Week 10 - Sunday
Food Menu

Today's Menu	What I Ate
1. Roast Beef Baked Potato Melted Cheese	
2. Protein Shake	
3. Turkey Sandwich	
4. Protein Shake	
5. Grilled Chicken Brown Rice Side Salad	
6. Yogurt or Protein Bar	

Week 10 – Sunday
Rest

a

Are you making every REP
and SET your best?

Week 11: Back-n-Forth

You will finish off this intense 12-week program with a new workout routine I have been using with great success.

Back-n-Forth is essentially a double Super Set. Just a double Super Set but feels like your fat is melting off! If you really want to fatigue a muscle group and make a stubborn body part change, this is the workout routine you can always count on for doing the job.

Back-n-Forth

- Complete the 1st exercise to failure.
- Complete the 2nd exercise to failure.
- Go back to the 1st exercise and go to failure.
- Go back to the 2nd exercise and go to failure.
- Rest up to 2-3 minutes before starting the next Back-n-Forth.

Example

Set 1: Leg Press to Leg Extension to Leg Press to Leg Extension.

Week 11

- Three workouts. Total body workouts.
- 4 Back-n-Forth Routines per workout.
- 8-15 reps per set.
- No rest during Back-n-Forth.
- Rest 2-3 minutes between sets.
- Keep eating clean +75% of the time.
- Drink lots of water. Do your cardio.

Week 11 - Monday
Food Menu

Today's Menu	What I Ate
1. Protein Shake	
2. Celery with Peanut Butter	
3. Grilled Chicken Sandwich	
4. Protein Shake	
5. Turkey Wrap	
6. Protein Shake or Bar	

Week 11: Back-n-Forth
Workout 1
-Total Body-

Exercise	Your Goal Reps x Weight		Your Set Reps x Weight	
1. BB Bench Press	10	30-60		
Lat Pulldown*	10	40-70		
BB Bench Press	10	30-60		
Lat Pulldown*	10	40-70		
2. BB Bench Press	10	30-60		
Lat Pulldown*	10	40-70		
BB Bench Press	10	30-60		
Lat Pulldown*	10	40-70		
3. Deadlifts	12	25-50		
Walking Lunges	F	10-20		
Deadlifts	12	25-50		
Walking Lunges	F	10-20		
4. DB Curls	12	10-20		
SkullKrushers	12	8-15		
DB Curls	12	10-20		
SkullKrushers	12	8-15		

Underhand Grip

Week 11 - Tuesday
Food Menu

Today's Menu	What I Ate
1. Protein Shake	
2. Baked Potato Cottage Cheese Turkey Breast	
3. Plain Yogurt with Fruit	
4. Protein Shake	
5. Lean Steak or Chicken Steamed Vegetables 2 Whole Wheat Bread	
6. Protein Shake or Bar	

Week 11 – Tuesday
Cardio Activity
20-40 Minutes

Week 11 - Wednesday
Food Menu

Today's Menu	What I Ate
1. 2-3 Egg Omelet 100% Whole Wheat Toast	
2. Protein Shake	
3. Grilled Chicken Sandwich Piece of Fruit or Vegetables	
4. Protein Shake	
5. Grilled Fish Steamed Vegetables Brown Rice	
6. Protein Shake or Bar	

Week 11: Back-n-Forth
Workout 2
-Total Body-

Exercise	Your Goal		Your Set	
	Reps x	Weight	Reps x	Weight
1. Rear Raise	10	5-10		
DB Press	10	10-20		
Rear Raise	10	5-10		
DB Press	10	10-20		
2. Incline Flys	10	10-15		
Incline Press	10	12-20		
Incline Flys	10	10-15		
Incline Press	10	12-20		
3. Leg Press	15	75-125		
Leg Extensions	15	40-60		
Leg Press	15	75-125		
Leg Extensions	15	40-60		
4. Leg Press	15	75-125		
Leg Extensions	15	40-60		
Leg Press	15	75-125		
Leg Extensions	15	40-60		

Week 11 – Thursday
Food Menu

Today's Menu	What I Ate
1. 2-3 Eggs 1-2 Pancakes	
2. Protein Shake	
3. Chili Whole Wheat Crackers Side Salad	
4. Protein Shake	
5. Pork Chops Steamed Vegetables Baked Potato	
6. Protein Shake or Bar	

Week 11 – Thursday
Rest

Week 11 - Friday
Food Menu

Today's Menu	What I Ate
1. Protein Shake	
2. Plain Yogurt Grape Nuts Banana	
3. Turkey Wrap	
4. Protein Shake	
5. Broiled Seafood Side Salad Sourdough Bread	
6. Protein Shake or Bar	

Week 11: Back-n-Forth
Workout 3
-Total Body-

Exercise	Your Goal Reps x Weight		Your Set Reps x Weight	
1. BB Squats	10	40-75		
Leg Curls	10	30-60		
BB Squats	10	40-75		
Leg Curls	10	30-60		
2. Pushdowns	10	20-30		
Tricep Ext.	10	10-20		
Pushdowns	10	20-30		
Tricep Ext.	10	10-20		
3. Pushdowns	10	20-30		
Tricep Ext.	10	10-20		
Pushdowns	10	20-30		
Tricep Ext.	10	10-20		
4. 2 DB Pullovers	8	10-20		
2 DB Rows	8	15-30		
2 DB Pullovers	8	10-20		
2 DB Rows	8	15-30		

Week 11 - Saturday
Food Menu

Today's Menu	What I Ate
1. Protein Shake	
2. Baked Potato Cottage Cheese Turkey Breast	
3. Tunafish Sandwich	
4. Protein Shake	
5. Grilled Chicken Salad	
6. Protein Shake or Bar	

Week 11 – Saturday
Cardio Activity
30-45 Minutes

Week 11 - Sunday
Food Menu

Today's Menu	What I Ate
1. Hard Boiled Eggs Fruit	
2. Protein Shake	
3. Pizza or Pasta!!!	
4. Protein Shake	
5. Cottage Cheese or (Eat a low carb food)	
6. Nothing!	

Week 11 – Sunday
Rest!

There is no such thing as a "quick fix". If you work hard, follow a proven plan and want it bad enough – the pay off will be AWESOME...guaranteed!

Week 12: Back-n-Forth

You made it! Last week and you are still here.

I BET YOU LOOK LIKE A NEW PERSON.
THE PERSON YOU HAVE ALWAYS WANTED TO LOOK LIKE!

If you can muster up the strength, you will be doing one more 5 day low-carb fat-melting week.

The final touches to your masterpiece – your new body.

Go get-em Tiger!

Week 12

- Two workouts.
- Total Body workouts.
- 1st workout early in the week.
- 2nd workout at end of low carb phase.
- Continue Back-n-Forth.
- Cardio 4 days.
- Drink lots of water!!

Week 12 – Monday
Food Menu

Today's Menu	What I Ate
1. 2-3 eggs	
2. Ham String Cheese	
3. Hot Dog(no bun) Pickles	
4. Skip Meal Diet Soda/Water	
5. Grilled Fish Lettuce/Cheese Salad	
6. Pumpkin Seeds	

Week 12: Back-n-Forth
Workout 1
-Total Body-

Exercise	Your Goal		Your Set	
	Reps x	Weight	Reps x	Weight
1. Rev Crunch	12	0		
Crunches	15	0-10		
Rev Crunch	12	0		
Crunch	15	0-10		
2. BB Press	15	25-40		
BB Curl	15	25-40		
BB Press	15	25-40		
BB Curl	15	25-40		
2. BB Press	8	25-40		
BB Curl	8	25-40		
BB Press	8	25-40		
BB Curl	8	25-40		
4. Leg Press	15	50-100		
Walking Lunges	F	10-20		
Leg Press	15	50-100		
Walking Lunges	F	10-20		

Week 12 – Tuesday
Food Menu

Today's Menu	What I Ate
1. Coffee/Tea/Water	
2. Bacon String Cheese	
3. Skip Meal Diet Soda/Water	
4. Steak Lettuce/Cheese Salad	
5. Fried Pork Rinds	
6. Skip Meal	

Week 12 - Tuesday
Cardio Activity
30-45 Minutes

Week 12 – Wednesday
Food Menu

Today's Menu	What I Ate
1. 2 Hard Boiled Eggs	
2. Celery w/Peanut Butter	
3. Chicken Breast	
4. Sugar Free Jello	
5. Shrimp Cocktail	
6. Diet Soda/Tea	

Week 12 – Wednesday
Cardio Activity
30-45 Minutes

Week 12 – Thursday
Food Menu

Today's Menu	What I Ate
1. Omelet w/Half&Half	
2. Diet/Coffee/Water	
3. No Bun Cheeseburger Pickles	
4. Cottage Cheese	
5. Grilled Tuna or Canned Tuna with Mayo & Pickles	
6. Diet Soda/Tea	

Week 12 - Thursday
Cardio Activity
30-45 Minutes

Week 12 – Friday
Food Menu

Today's Menu	What I Ate
1. Ham & Eggs	
2. Fried Pork Rinds	
3. Grilled Chicken Salad	
4. Cheese Olives	
5. *AFTER YOUR WORKOUT* Protein Shake w/Carbs	
6. Whatever you want- Pig out!!!!	

Week 12: Back-n-Forth
Workout 2
-Total Body-

Exercise	Your Goal Reps x Weight		Your Set Reps x Weight	
. DB Bench Press	10	15-30		
2 DB Rows	10	15-30		
DB Bench Press	10	15-30		
2 DB Rows	10	15-30		
. DB Bench	10	15-30		
2 DB Rows	10	15-30		
DB Bench	10	15-30		
2 DB Rows	10	15-30		
. Leg Extensions	15	25-50		
Leg Curls	8	25-50		
Leg Extensions	15	25-50		
Leg Curls	8	25-50		
. Leg Extensions	15	25-50		
Leg Curls	8	25-50		
Leg Extensions	15	25-50		
Leg Curls	8	25-50		

Week 12 – Saturday
Food Menu

Today's Menu	What I Ate
1. Bowl of Cereal	
2. Protein Shake	
3. Pizza	
4. Protein Shake	
5. Pasta Meal	
6. Glass of Wine or Beer or Juice	

Week 12 – Saturday
Rest!

Now What?

The best thing to do after completing *Weight Training Workouts and Diet Plan that Work* is to take a few days off to let your body and brain rest. You do not want to over-train.

Now it's time to start the program over again. You will be a lot stronger and fit. The exercises will be more comfortable. You will make amazing progress towards your ideal health and body.

DO NOT FOLLOW THE LOW CARBS WEEKS THE 2ND TIME THROUGH THE PROGRAM. Using low carbs too often diminishes the positive effect to your body and is hard to sustain. Use low carb weeks sparingly after the first time through the 12 weeks. One week every 2-3 months is usually enough. Substitute a different food menu for the low carb weeks but follow the same workouts.

If you find some exercises that personally work better for you, replace them with the exercises you do not like. Just remember not to get stuck in a rut of using the same exercises or workouts too often. Your results will diminish if you do not use variety.

Good Luck, IT WORKS!

James Orvis
james@weighttrainingworkouts.com
www.weighttrainingworkouts.com

234

Part II
The Best Weight Training Exercises

Abs

Ab Bench Crunches

Muscles Used: Abs
Starting Weight: 0-10

- Set or use a bench with 10-30 degree decline.
- Lock-in legs.
- Place hands across chest.
- Do not put your hands behind your head, you can pull on your neck and spine.
- Slowly lower your body, keeping your back slightly rounded.
- Lower upper body until nearing parallel to the floor. *Do not go too low until you are strong enough!*
- Keep abs tight throughout movement.
- Return to starting position, stopping just before you are straight up to keep tension on the abs.
- Repeat until set is complete

Ab Bench Crunches

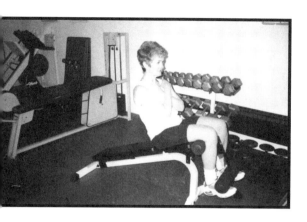

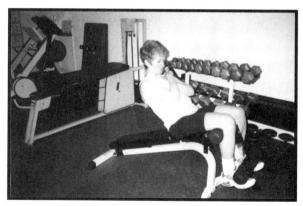

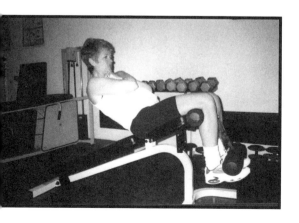

Abs

Ball Crunches

Muscles Used: Abs
Starting Weight: 0-10

- Lie on the ball with your knees bent at about a 90-degree angle. Make sure your feet are securely on the floor, wide enough to stabilize your upper body.
- *Make sure you are careful the first few times you perform ball crunches. You could be unstable and roll off the ball, so do not have any equipment around you that could be potentially dangerous.*
- Put your hands across your chest.
- Slowly curl up keeping your abs tight.
- Exhale as you curl up.
- Curl up about 30 degrees.
- Slowly lower until you feel a nice stretch in your abs.
- Inhale as you lower.
- Repeat until set is complete.
- Only lower as far as you feel comfortable. *Make sure you do not go too far back until your abs and lower back are strong enough!* The ball works super for abs because you can lower past parallel to the floor. Your abs work approximately 30 degrees forward <u>and</u> 30 degrees backwards. When you perform all your ab exercises on a flat surface, you are only doing half the range of motion. The ball helps you train the abs through their full range.
- TIP: Add a weight plate or dumbbell across your chest when you need more resistance.

Abs

Ball Crunches

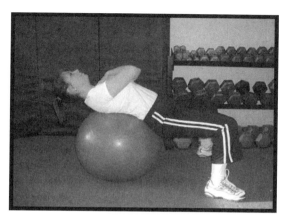

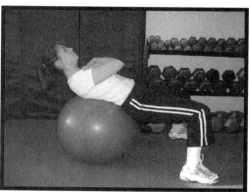

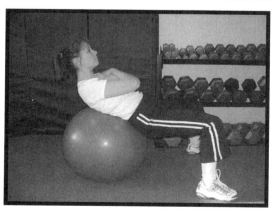

Abs

Ball V-Ups

Muscles Used: Lower Abs, Upper Abs
Starting Weight: 0 lbs.

- Lie on the floor placing the ball between your knees and lower legs. Hands across you chest.
- Slowly lift up your upper body <u>and</u> legs at the same time.
- Exhale as you lift.
- Lift you upper body about 30 degrees while pulling your legs toward your chest area, squeezing your abs tight.
- Pause on the top position.
- Slowly lower to starting position.
- Inhale while lowering.
- Stop right before your shoulders and feet touch the floor.
- This keeps constant tension on your abs.
- Repeat until set is complete.
- TIP: If the exercise is too hard to perform or you become fatigued quickly, keep your lower body on the floor and just curl up your legs. Concentrate on you lower abs doing the work.

Ball V-Ups

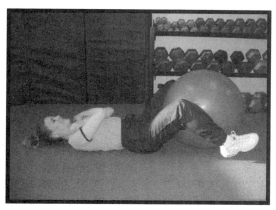

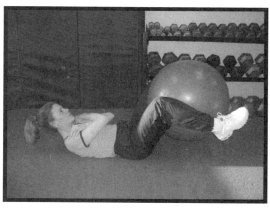

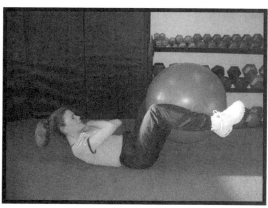

Abs

Crunches

Muscles Used: Abs
Starting Weight: 0-10

- Lie on your back.
- Knees bent, feet on the floor.
- Put hands across your chest.
  Do not put your hands behind your head.
- Curl up about 30-degrees. Do not go up all the way.
- Hold for a second.
- Slowly lower until right before your shoulders fully touch the floor. This will keep tension on your abs.
- Repeat until set is complete.
- TIP: Keep your stomach flexed during the entire exercise- *"like you are getting ready for someone to punch you in the stomach."*
- TIP: When adding weight for resistance, hold a weight plate or a dumbbell across your chest.

Crunches

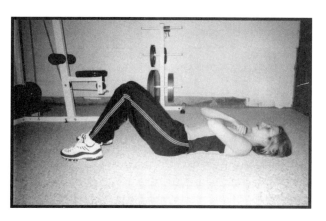

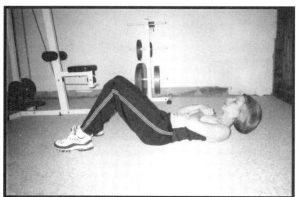

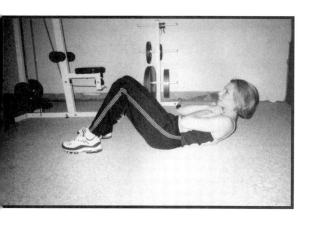

Abs

Reverse Crunches

Muscles Used: Lower Abs
Starting Weight: 0

- Set bench at approximately a 30-degree decline.
- Lay on your back, head at the top of the bench. Make sure your head is flat on the bench.
- Hang on to the top of the bench. This can be the hardest part of the exercise in the beginning. Just grab onto whatever you can, it will become easier.
- Curl up your legs as far as you feel comfortable, knees bent.
- Pause for a second at the top.
- Slowly lower legs.
- Lower as far as you feel comfortable. Your lower back and abs will become stronger with this exercise.
- Repeat until set is complete.
- TIP: Use a spotter to help lift your legs.
- TIP: If your lower back is weak, substitute another ab exercise until you feel strong enough to perform reverse crunches.

Reverse Crunches

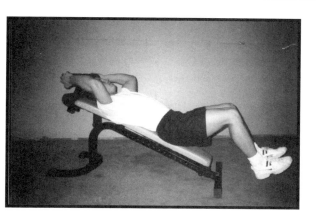

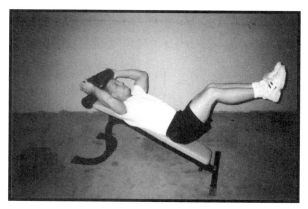

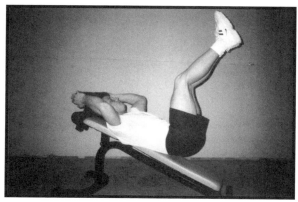

Abs

Wood Chop

Muscles Used: Abs, Entire Mid-Section
Starting Weight: 10-20 lbs.

- Use the rope attachment on a low pulley.
- Stand with you with feet shoulder width apart or wider so you have stability.
- Make sure you are far enough away from the pulley, 1 to 2 feet, so you can perform the exercise through the full range of motion.
- Grasp both ends of the rope together, with your palms facing down.
- With your arms slightly bent, pull up rope diagonally and twist body at the same time.
- *Concentrate on your mid-section pulling the weight up, not your arms.*
- Exhale when pulling up.
- Stop when you are fully extended.
- Slowly lower the weight, keeping your mid-section tight all the way to the starting position.
- Inhale while lowering the weight.
- Repeat until set is complete.
- TIP: This is a very mental exercise! To have to think about your entire midsection doing the work, not your arms.
- TIP: Remember to turn around and do your other side.

Wood Chop

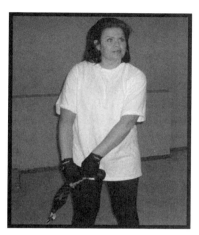

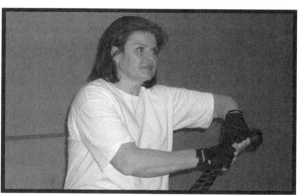

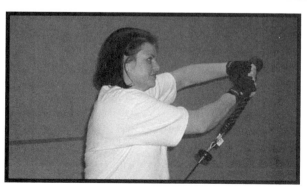

Back

Lat Pulldown - Wide Grip

Muscles Used: Upper & Mid Back, Biceps
Starting Weight: 40-70 lbs.

- Grasp the straight bar with an overhand grip, palms facing away from you.
- Hands 2-3 inches wider than your shoulders. Do not go too wide, this can put undue stress on your shoulders.
- Holding bar, sit down and lock knees under pad. Adjust height of pad if needed.
- *Lean back, with chest out during entire movement.*
- First movement should be pulling your shoulder blades back and together. *Think of someone putting a finger between your shoulder blades and you trying to squeeze their finger.*
- Pull the bar all the way down to the mid-upper chest area, concentrating on your upper back.
- Elbows half way between your sides and straight out.
- Stop for a second, then slowly resist the bar all the way up. Remember to keep your chest out and shoulders back through the entire movement.
- Keep back muscles tight.
- Return the bar all the way up until you feel a slight stretch in your mid-upper back muscles.
- Repeat until set is complete.

Back

Lat Pulldown - Wide Grip

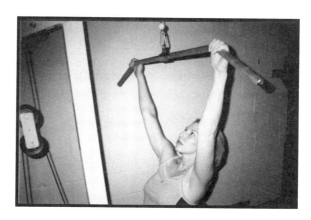

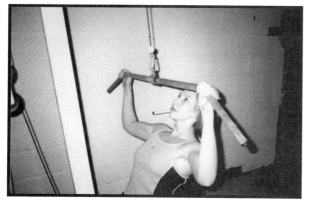

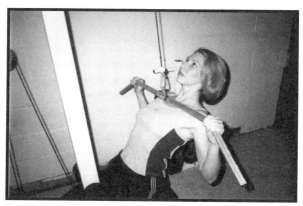

Back

Lat Pulldown – Underhand Grip

Muscles Used: Mid Back, Biceps
Starting Weight: 40-70 lbs.

Same as Lat Pulldown - Wide Grip except:
- Underhand grip with palms facing you.
- Hands approximately 1 –2 feet apart.
- Pull to low-mid chest area.
- Elbows along the sides of your body.

Lat Pulldown – Underhand Grip

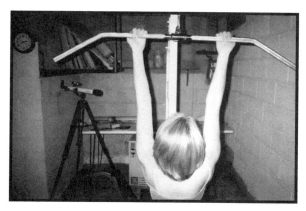

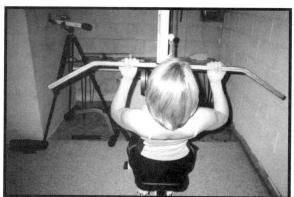

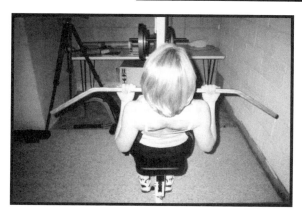

Back

Lat Pulldown - Triangle Bar

Muscles Used: Mid-Outer Back, Biceps
Starting Weight: 40-70 lbs.

Same as Lat Pulldown - Wide Grip except:

- Use the Triangle Bar (also called the V-Bar).
- Palms facing each other.
- Pull to mid-chest.
- Elbows along the sides of your body.
- Concentrate on mid and outer sides of back.

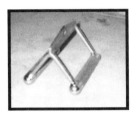

Triangle Bar

Back

Lat Pulldown - Triangle Bar

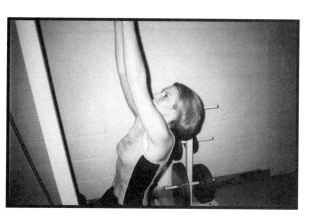

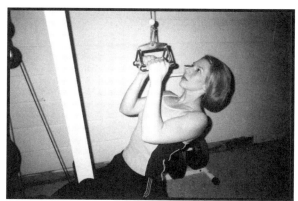

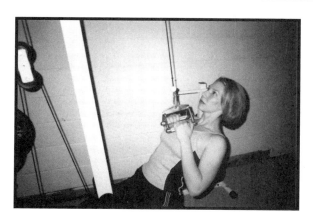

Back

Dumbbell Pullovers

Muscles Used: Back, Triceps, Chest
Starting Weight: 15-25 lbs.

- Lay on the bench with your feet on the floor or bench.
- Your head at the end of the bench. Make sure your head is supported on the bench.
- Grasp a dumbbell on the inside end with your palms flat, overlapping each other securely. See illustration below.
- Keep elbows in and pointed forward, towards your feet.
- Slowly lower the dumbbell behind your head
- Keep your muscles tight!
- Lower until upper arms are beside your head and lower arms are bent.
- Feel a good stretch in your abs, back and triceps. Do not go too far down right away. If your shoulders start to feel weak, stop. You will become stronger and more flexible.
- <u>Slowly pull up with your elbows, not your hands</u>. This will emphasize your back muscles.
- Straighten your arms towards the top of movement.
- Stop when the dumbbell is straight over your chest/shoulder area.
- Repeat until set is complete.

254

Dumbbell Pullovers

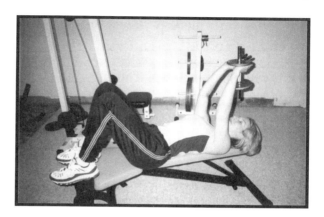

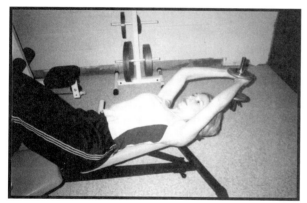

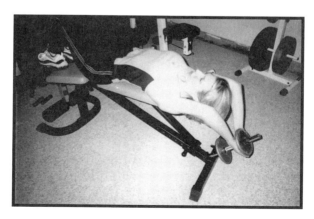

Back

2 Dumbbell Pullovers

Muscles Used: Back, Triceps, Chest
Starting Weight: 5-15 lbs.

- Lay on the bench with your feet on the floor or the bench.
- Your head at the end of the bench. Make sure your head is supported on the bench.
- Grasp 2 dumbbells. Hold straight up over your shoulder area.
- Palms facing each other.
- Keep elbows in and pointed forward, towards your feet.
- Slowly lower the dumbbells behind your head.
- Keep your muscles tight!
- Lower until upper arms are beside your head and lower arms are bent.
- Feel a good stretch in your abs, back and triceps.
- Do not go too far down right away. If your shoulders start to feel weak, stop. You will become stronger and more flexible.
- Slowly pull up with your elbows, not your hands. This will emphasize your back muscles.
- Straighten your arms towards the top of movement.
- Stop when the dumbbells is straight over your chest/shoulder area.
- Repeat until set is complete.

Back

2 Dumbbell Rows

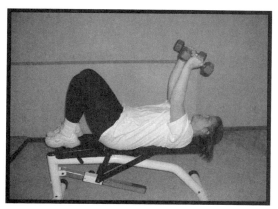

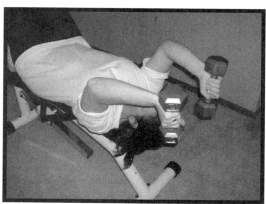

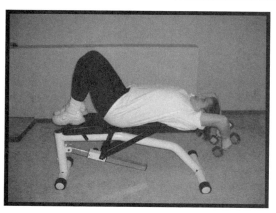

Back

2 Dumbbell Rows

Muscles Used: Mid Back, Upper and Lower Back, Biceps
Starting Weight: 10-20 lbs.

- Sit on the end of a bench.
- Feet close together.
- Grasp 2 dumbbells.
- Bend over keeping your back flat and your head up.
- *Make sure to keep your head up or in the neutral position during the entire exercise. This will keep your back flat. If you look down your back will start to round, which will put undue stress on your lower back.*
- Keeping head up and chest out, pull up dumbbells squeezing your shoulder blades together.
- Keep your elbows in, pulling along sides of your body.
- Exhale as you pull up the dumbbells.
- Squeeze you shoulder blades together on the top, feeling your back do the work.
- Slowly lower the weight, keeping your head up and back flat.
- Inhale on the lowering phase.
- TIP: Move your upper body with the motion. When your pulling the weight up, move your upper body up with the weight stopping at about a 70 degree angle to the floor. When lowering the weight, lower your upper body with the weight. This will help keep stress off your lower back.

Back

2 Dumbbell Rows

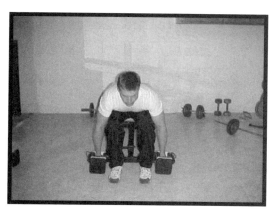

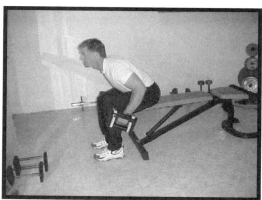

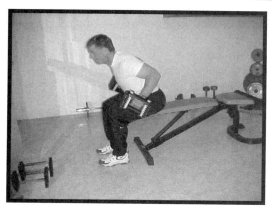

Biceps

Barbell Curls

Muscles Used: Biceps
Starting Weight: 20-30 lbs.

- Standing, feet shoulder width apart.
- Knees slightly bent.
- Palms forward, slightly wider than shoulder width apart.
- Elbows touching your sides.
- Curl the weight up towards your shoulders/chin area until biceps are fully contracted.
- Look straight ahead and do not to arch your back during lifting phase.
- Slowly lower the weight.
- Stop right before your elbows lock out.
- Repeat until set is complete.

Barbell Curls

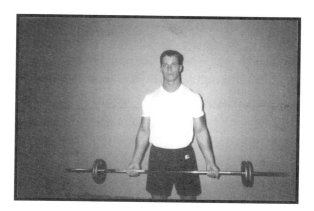

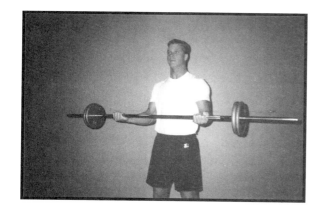

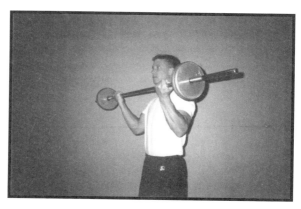

Biceps

Cable Curls

Muscles Used: Biceps
Starting Weight: 15-30 lbs.

- Stand facing the low pulley machine.
- 1-2 feet away from the pulley.
- Grasp bar, palms up, about shoulder width apart.
- You can also use the rope attachment. Your palms will be facing each when using the rope.
- Keep your elbows *stuck* at your sides during entire movement.
- Curl up weight concentrating on your biceps doing the work.
- Keep your back straight.
- Exhale as you lift the weight.
- Slowly lower the weight to starting position, letting the biceps do all the work.
- Stop right before your elbows lock out. This will keep constant tension on you biceps and is easy on your joints.
- Inhale as you lower the weight.
- Repeat until set is complete.

Biceps

Cable Curls

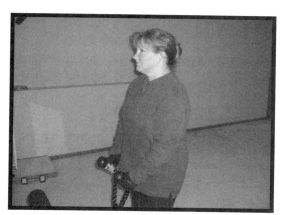

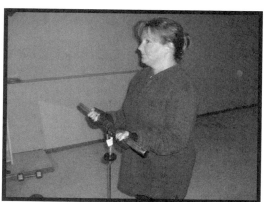

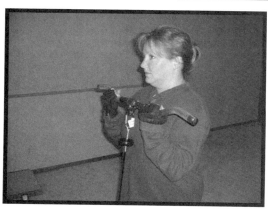

Biceps

Dumbbell Curls

Muscles Used: Biceps
Starting Weight: 10-20 lbs.

- Seated, feet firmly on the floor.
- Back straight.
- Dumbbells hanging at your sides.
- Palms facing each other.
- Elbows pressed against your sides (elbows do not move).
- Curl dumbbells at the same time towards your shoulders, rotating palms so they are facing up when biceps are fully contracted.
- Slowly lower weight, rotating palms back so they are facing each other again at the bottom.
- Stop right before elbows lock out.
- Repeat until set is complete.

Biceps

Dumbbell Curls

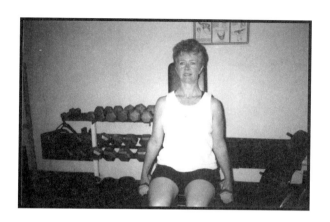

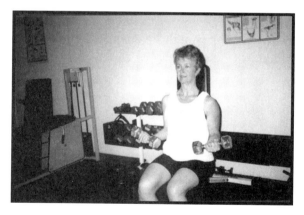

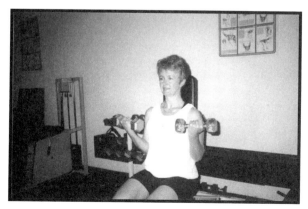

Biceps

Hammer Curls

Muscles Used: Outer Biceps
Starting Weight: 8-15 lbs.

- Seated, feet firmly on the floor.
- Back straight.
- Dumbbells hanging at your sides.
- Palms facing each other.
- Elbows pressed against your sides.
- Elbows do not move during entire movement.
- Curl dumbbells at the same time towards your shoulders, keeping your palms facing each other.
- Exhale as you lift the weight.
- Slowly lower weight to starting position.
- Stop right before elbows lock out.
- Inhale as you lower the weight.
- Repeat until set is complete.

Biceps

Hammer Curls

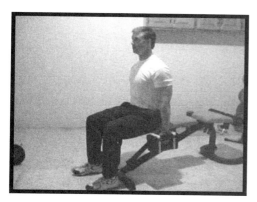

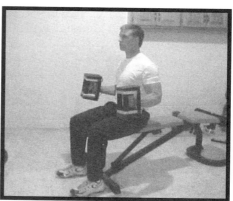

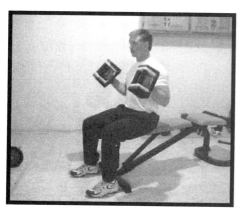

267

Biceps

Incline Curls

Muscles Used: Lower Biceps
Starting Weight: 8-15 lbs.

- Set or use a bench at a 70-80 degree angle.
- Seated, feet firmly on the floor or locked in place.
- Back flat against the bench.
- You can keep your head up (off the bench) if it is more comfortable.
- Dumbbells hanging at your sides.
- Palms facing each other.
- Elbows pressed against your sides.
- Elbows do not move during entire movement.
- Curl dumbbells at the same time towards your shoulders, turning you palms up during the movement.
- Exhale as you lift the weight.
- Slowly lower weight to starting position.
- Turning your palms back to facing each other.
- Stop right before elbows lock out.
- Inhale as you lower the weight.
- Repeat until set is complete.
- TIP: When your biceps become fatigued, you can keep your palms up the entire movement. This should help you complete a couple extra reps.

Incline Curls

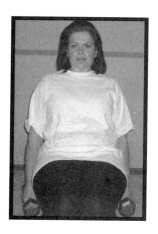

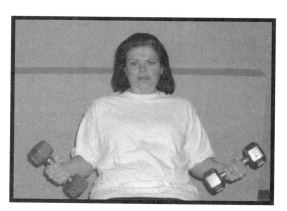

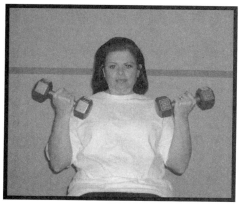

Chest

Barbell Bench Press

Muscles Used: Chest, Shoulders, Triceps
Starting Weight: 30-60 lbs.

- Lay flat on the bench with your feet on the floor or bench, keeping your lower back flat.
- Grasp barbell, palms facing forward, slightly wider than shoulder width apart. You can experiment with your hand position but do not go too wide or narrow because this can put undue stress on your shoulders.
- Slowly lower the bar to your mid-chest with elbows straight out to the sides.
- Lightly touch middle of the chest. Do not bounce! Upper and lower arms should be at a right angle.
- Feel a stretch in your chest and mentally push up with your chest muscles.
- Stop right before you lock out on top.
- Repeat until set is complete.
- TIP: Make sure to use a spotter with heavy weights.

Chest

Barbell Bench Press

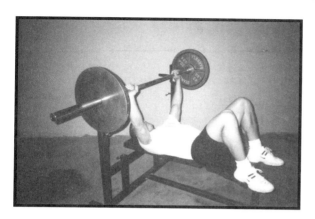

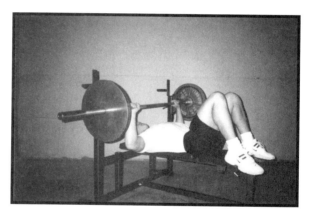

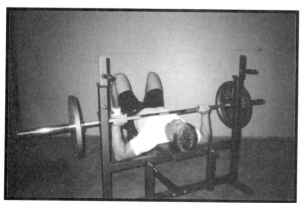

Chest

Dumbbell Bench Press

Muscles Used: Chest, Shoulders, Triceps
Starting Weight: 10-20 lbs.

- Lay flat on the bench with your feet on the floor or bench, keeping your lower back flat.
- Bring dumbbells to the starting position with your palms facing forward towards your feet.
- Slowly lower dumbbells, elbows straight out to the sides.
- Lower until you feel a good stretch in your chest and your arms are at about a 90-degree angle.
- If your front shoulders start to pull too much, stop. *You will become stronger and more flexible with practice.*
- Push straight up.
- Stop right before you lock out on top.
- Repeat until set is complete.

Chest

Dumbbell Bench Press

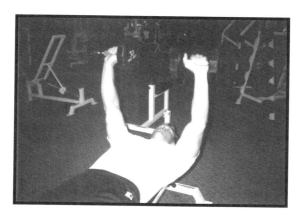

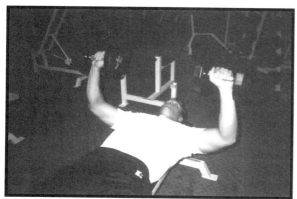

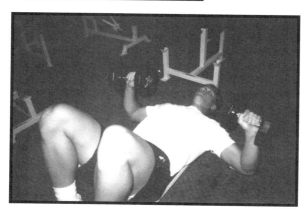

Chest

Incline Dumbbell Bench Press

Muscles Used: Upper Chest, Shoulders, Triceps
Starting Weight: 8-20 lbs.

- Set or use a bench with approximately a 45-degree incline.
- Feet on floor and lower back pushed against the backrest.
- Bring dumbbells to the starting position with your palms facing forward towards your feet.
- Slowly lower dumbbells, elbows straight out to the sides.
- Lower until you feel a good stretch in your upper chest and your arms are at about a 90-degree angle. If your front shoulders start to pull too much, stop.
- *You will become stronger and more flexible with practice.*
- Push straight up.
- Stop right before your elbows lock out on top.
- Repeat until set is complete.

Incline Dumbbell Bench Press

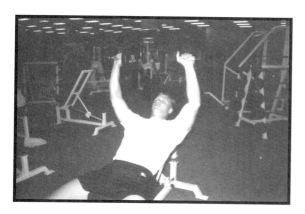

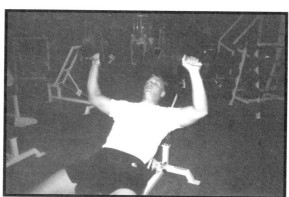

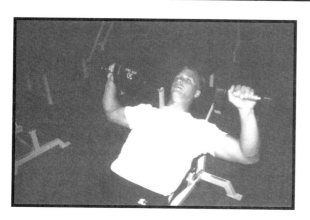

Chest

Incline Flys

Muscles Used: Upper Chest
Starting Weight: 8-15 lbs.

- Lie on an incline bench, feet on the floor.
- Bench should be about a 45-degree angle.
- Bring the dumbbells to the starting position.
- Palms facing forward.
- *Keep elbows slightly bent during the movement.*
- Slowly lower dumbbells straight out to your sides.
- *Let gravity pull the weight down.*
- Keep your chest muscles tight.
- Lower until you feel a stretch in your chest muscles.
- Make sure you stop lowering the weight if you start to feel your front shoulders pulling too much.
- *Mentally pull up with your chest, not concentrating on your arms.*
- Keep chest flexed throughout movement, especially the top part of the exercise.
- Repeat until set is complete.
- TIP: The movement should be in an arc, with gravity pulling the dumbbells down. Keep your arms about the same angle throughout the movement, this is not a pressing movement.

Incline Flys

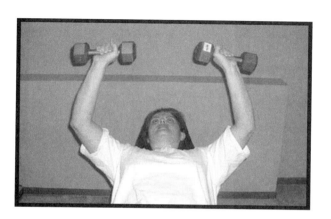

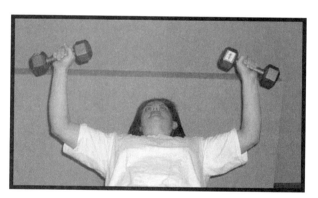

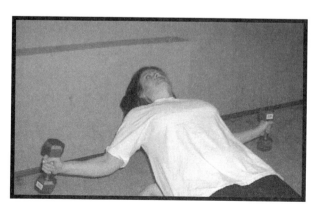

Chest

Twisting Dumbbell Bench Press

Muscles Used: Chest, Shoulders, Triceps
Starting Weight: 10-20 lbs.

- Grasp dumbbells and lie on a flat bench.
- Feet on the floor or bench, back flat.
- Start at the bottom position with your palms facing each other.
- *Push the dumbbells up, at the same time pushing your elbows back and up, turning your palms forward so they are facing your feet.*
- Stop right before your elbows lock out.
- Exhale as you lift the weight.
- Slowly lower the weight to starting position, turning your palms in and pulling your elbows in at the same time.
- Inhale as you lower the weight.
- Repeat until set is complete.
- TIP: Concentrate on your chest muscles during the entire exercise, not your arms.
- TIP: Practice with light weights until you feel comfortable with the exercise and can feel you chest doing the work. This exercise may take a little time to perfect the form and feeling your chest do all the work.

Twisting Dumbbell Bench Press

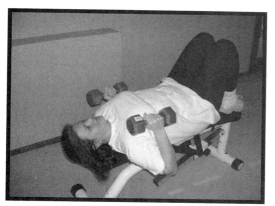

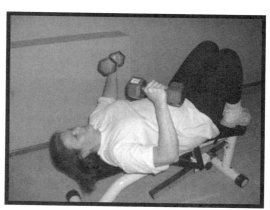

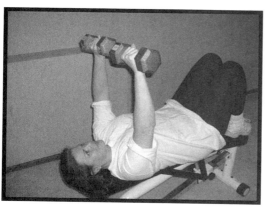

Legs

Barbell Squats

Muscles Used: Quads, Glutes, Hamstrings
Starting Weight: 45-75 lbs.

- Tip - Use a squat rack or a spotter if available.
- Place barbell on your upper back, not on your neck. Use a bar pad if available.
- Feet shoulder width apart, toes slightly pointed out about 10 degrees.
- Focus eyes straight ahead during entire movement.
- Slowly lower, bending at the knees. Think of sitting down in a chair.
- Your hips and butt go back. Knees straight over your feet.
- Knees behind your feet. If your knees are going in front of your feet too much, it puts undue stress on your knees. Make sure your rear end is going out.
- Keep your back straight. Your back will be *flat* but at a 70-80 degree angle to the floor.
- Stop when your quads become parallel to the floor. This is your goal, but start by only lowering a short distance until you learn the exercise and become stronger.
- Push straight up under control.
- Breath out when you are half way up in the return phase.
- Stop right before your knees lock out.
- Repeat until set is complete.
- TIP: If your lower back starts to develop a dull throb, stop and rest. Your lower back will probably be the first muscles to become tired, but will become stronger with practice.

280

Barbell Squats

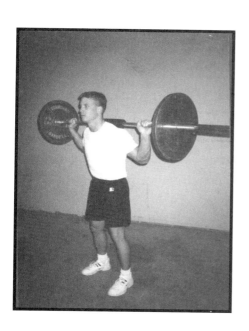

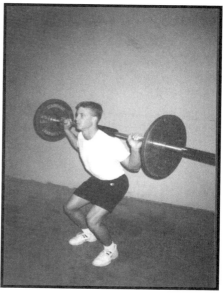

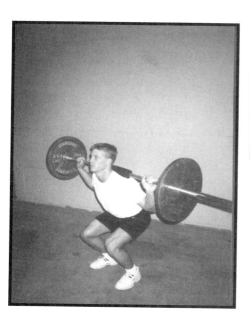

Legs

Dumbbell Squats

Muscles Used: Quads, Glutes, Hamstrings
Starting Weight: 10-20lbs.

- Grasp dumbbells, palms facing each other at your sides.
- Feet shoulder width apart or a little narrower so the dumbbells do not get in the way. Toes slightly pointed out 10 degrees.
- Focus eyes straight ahead during entire movement.
- Slowly lower, bending at the knees. Think of sitting in a chair.
- Your hips and butt go back. Knees straight over your feet.
- Knees behind your feet. If your knees are going in front of your feet too much, it puts undue stress on your knees. Make sure your rear end is going out.
- Keep your back straight. Your back will be *flat* but will be at a 70-80 degree angle to the floor.
- Stop when your quads become parallel to the floor..
- Push straight up under control.
- Breath out when you are half way up in the return phase.
- Stop right before your knees lock out.
- Repeat until set is complete.
- TIP: If your heels start to lift up while lowering, use small weight plates, 5 or 10 lbs. under your heels to help stabilize your body.

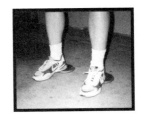

Dumbbell Squats

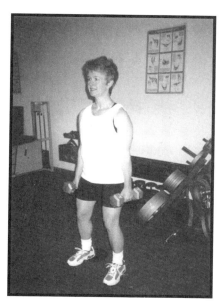

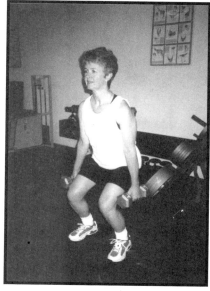

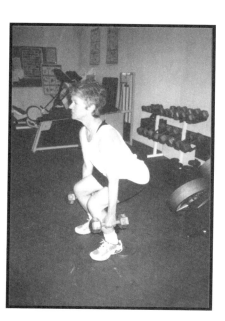

Legs

Deadlifts

Muscles Used: Hamstrings, Glutes, Lower Back
Starting Weight: 20-45 lbs.

- Grasp barbell, palms facing you.
- Hands shoulder width apart.
- Feet straight-ahead, about a foot apart.
- Hold barbell with arms straight, at mid thigh.
- Keep back flat, shoulders back, chest out and knees slightly bent throughout movement.
- Lower bar, right in front of your body, until about mid-shin level. *Do not go too far down, only until it feels comfortable.*
- Hips and rear end go back, bending at the waist.
- Feel a stretch in your hamstrings.
- Pull up to the starting position,
- Concentrate on your hamstrings, not your back.
- Repeat until set is complete.
- TIP: Remember to keep your back flat. Do not round your back. Keep your head in the neutral position.
- TIP: Do not use too heavy of weights.

Deadlifts

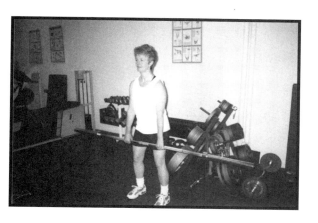

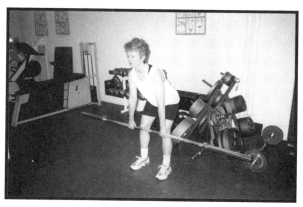

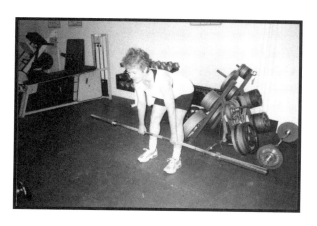

Legs

Calf Raises

Muscles Used: Calf
Starting Weight: 75-100 lbs.

- Do calf raises on the Leg Press Machine.
- Place balls of feet on the edge of the platform, knees relatively straight.
- Push up as far as possible until you feel a stretch at the top of the movement.
- Slowly lower heels until you feel a good stretch in your calves.
- Repeat until set is complete.
- TIP: If you don't have access to the Leg Press, you can do calf raises on the stairs, a calf block or any calf machine. There are many excellent types of machines at health clubs and gyms. Use the same form on all calf exercises.

Calf Raises

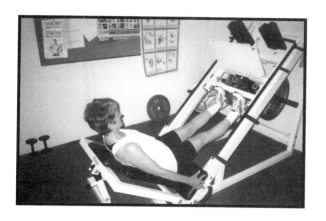

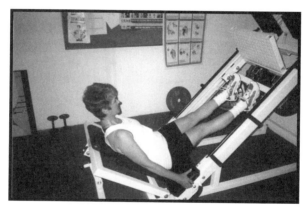

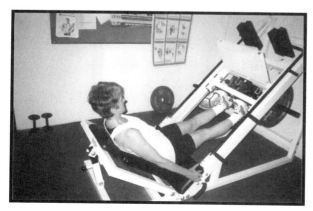

Legs

Leg Extensions

Muscles Used: Quads
Starting Weight: 30-50 lbs.

- Sit on the Leg Extension machine.
- Back firmly against the back pad.
- Back of knee against pad. Adjust the machine if needed.
- Lower leg pad on lower shin. Adjust the machine if needed.
- Slowly raise the weight until thigh is fully flexed and hold for a second, feeling your quads flex.
- *Do not hyperextend knees by raising the weight too fast.*
- Slowly lower.
- Stop before your lower leg goes past a 90-degree angle. By doing this, it keeps undue pressure off your knees.
- Repeat set until complete.

Leg Extensions

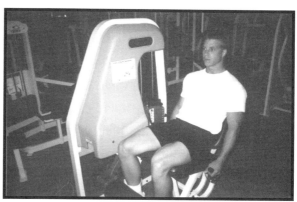

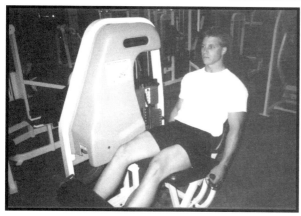

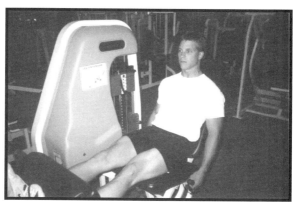

Legs

Leg Curls

Muscles Used: Hamstrings
Starting Weight: 30-50 lbs.

- Lie face down on the Leg Curl machine.
- Knees right behind the thigh pad.
- Lower leg pad above your heels.
- Grab handles or the bench.
- Pull the weight up slowly, especially the first 2-3 inches. This will make the hamstrings do the work.
- Stop when your feet are straight up or close to your rear end.
- *Keep your hips in contact with the bench at all times.*
- Slowly lower the weight.
- Stop right before your knees lock out.
- Repeat until set is complete.

Legs

Leg Curls

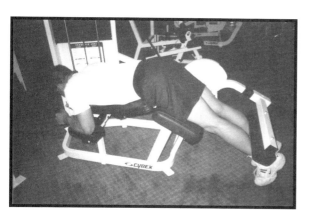

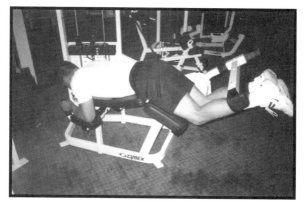

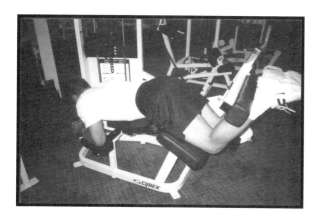

Legs

Leg Press

Muscles Used: Quads, Hamstrings, Glutes
Starting Weight: 75-125 lbs.

- Adjust the backrest so it is near the middle setting.
- Higher up if you are small person, lower if you are larger.
- Back and glutes firmly against the pads.
- Place your feet on top half of the platform.
- Feet shoulder width apart.
- Toes *slightly* pointed out about 10-degrees.
- Grasp handles, push up platform and unlock weights.
- Slowly lower knees towards your chest.
- When your legs go slightly past 90-degrees, stop. Make sure your butt does not start to lift up. If it does, stop, you have gone too far. That can put undue stress on your back.
- Slowly push the weights up, through your heels. This will take pressure off your knees.
- Stop right before your knees lock out.
- Repeat until set is complete.
- TIP: Find out how much the Leg Press weighs before you add weight. Every machine is different.
- TIP: Verticle and Horizontal Leg Press machines also work well. Use the same form as above.

Legs

Leg Press

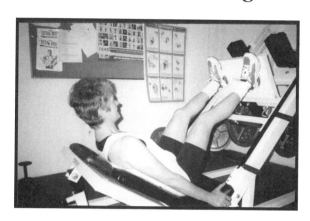

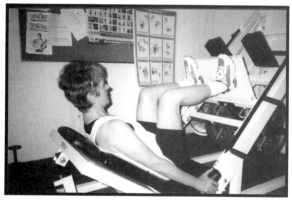

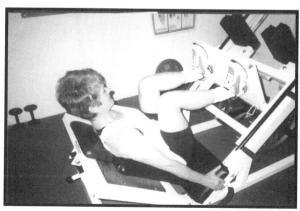

Legs

Stationary Lunges

Muscles Used: Glutes, Hamstrings, Quads
Starting Weight: 0 Lbs

- You exercise one leg at a time.
- Grasp a bench, machine, etc., something stable.
- Step forward with lead leg.
- Slowly lower straight down, keeping your back flat.
- Do not lean forward.
- Bend knee of lead leg until it reaches close to 90-degree angle. In the beginning, only bend your front knee as far as you feel comfortable.
- Keep knee over and behind lead foot. Make sure you are going straight up and down. Do not lean forward.
- Knee of back leg should be a few inches off the floor.
- Push straight up.
- Stop right before your front knee locks out.
- Repeat until set is complete.
- Switch lead leg.
- TIP: When you become stronger you can do lunges without holding on to a stable object. After that becomes too easy, you can add dumbbells in each hand for more resistance.

Stationary Lunges

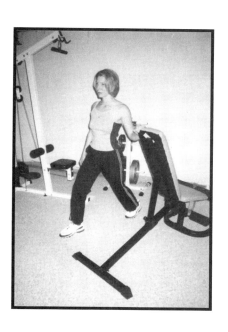

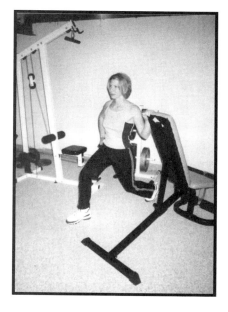

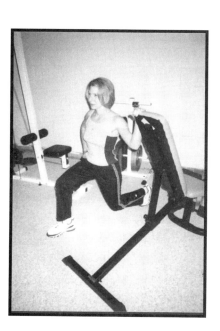

Legs

Walking Lunges

Muscles Used: Glutes, Hamstrings, Quads
Starting Weight: 5-15 lbs.

- Grasp dumbbells.
- Stand straight up with the dumbbells hanging at your sides.
- Feet hip-width width apart and toes pointed straight ahead.
- Take a step forward. *Make sure you step forward easy, don't come down hard on your front foot.*
- Keep your upper body upright and head looking straight ahead.
- Bend your lead leg so your upper leg is parallel to the ground.
- *Keep your lead knee directly over your foot when lowering. Do not lean forward and let your knee drift in front of your foot. This is hard on your knees.*
- Inhale as you lower.
- Push up while bring your back leg forward, just like you are walking.
- Exhale as you push up.
- Take a step forward. *Make sure you step forward easy, don't come down hard on your front foot.*
- Repeat until your legs are fatigued.
- TIP: If you ever start to lose you balance, STOP!
  Walking Lunges are a great exercise but
  require perfect form for safety.
- TIP: If you are new to lunges, make sure you start with Stationary Lunges until you feel comfortable. Then start using Walking Lunges with very light weights!

Walking Lunges

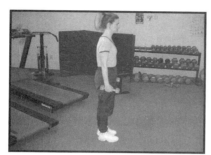

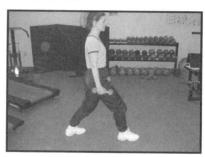

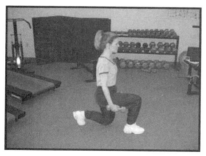

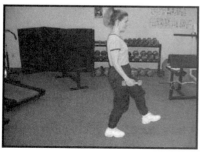

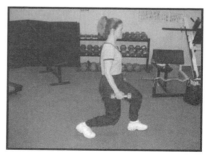

Shoulders

Barbell Press

Muscles Used: Shoulders, Triceps, Upper Back
Starting Weight: 20-40 lbs.

- Stand with feet shoulder width apart.
- Keep knees slightly bent.
- Bring barbell to the starting position.
- Palms forward, just slightly wider than shoulder width apart.
- Push barbell straight up in front of your face.
- Be sure to look straight ahead during entire movement, this will keep your back as straight as possible.
- Stop right before elbows lock out.
- *Slowly lower barbell to chin/neck level.*
- Keeps tension on your shoulders.
- Repeat until set is complete.
- TIP: Use a spotter if available.

Shoulders
Barbell Press

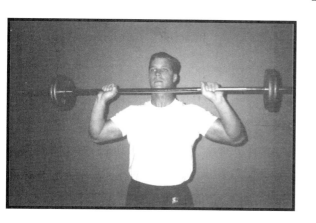

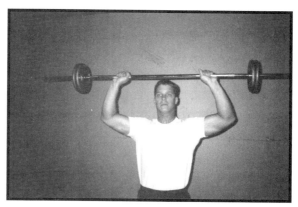

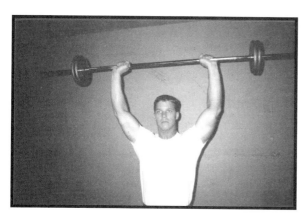

Shoulders

Dumbbell Press

Muscles Used: Shoulders, Triceps
Starting Weight: 8-15 lbs.

- Seated, back flat against bench, feet firmly on the floor.
- Grasp dumbbells.
- Bring dumbbells to starting position, palms facing forward.
- Arms should be at a right angle.
- Push straight up, stopping right before your elbows lock out.
- Make sure to keep your back straight. Keep it pressed against the backrest.
- Slowly lower.
- Stop when dumbbells are in line with your ears, arms at a right angle. It keeps tension on your shoulders.
- Repeat until set is complete.

Shoulders
Dumbbell Press

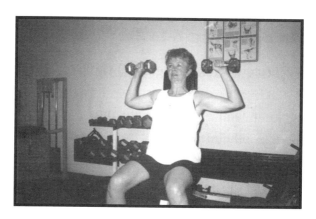

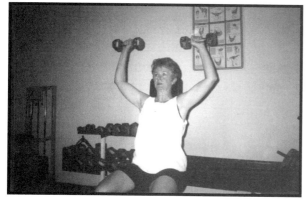

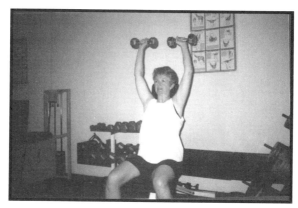

Shoulders

Front Raise

Muscles Used: Front Shoulders, Upper Back
Starting Weight: 3-10 lbs.

- Stand with your feet shoulder width apart or a little wider.
- Grasp 2 dumbbells with your palms facing you.
- Keep your elbows slightly bent during the entire movement.
- Raise the dumbbells directly in front of you.
- Raise to head level.
- Exhale as you lift the dumbbells.
- Keep you back flat. Don't arch your back.
- *Concentrate on your shoulders and upper back lifting the weights, not your arms.*
- Slowly lower the dumbbells, stopping before the weights are all the way down. This will keep constant tension on the muscles.
- Inhale as you lower.
- Repeat until set is complete.

Shoulders

Front Raise

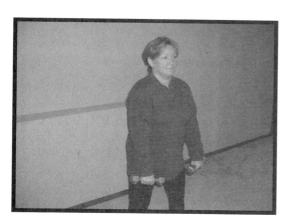

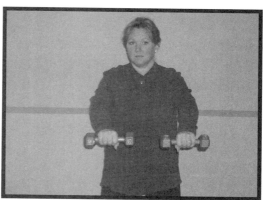

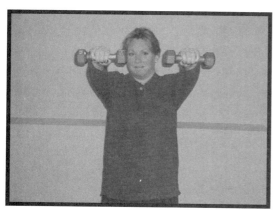

Shoulders

Rear Raise

Muscles Used: Rear Shoulders, Upper Back
Starting Weight: 3-10 lbs.

- Sit on the end of a flat bench.
- Feet close together.
- Grasp 2 dumbbells, palms facing each other.
- Bend over, keeping your back flat and your head up.
- *Try to look forward during entire movement. This will keep your back flat. You do not want it to round. This will happen if you start to look down, putting your back in an unsafe position.*
- Keeping your elbows slightly bent, raise your arms straight out to the sides like you are flying.
- The dumbbells should be in line with your head.
- Raise the weights as high as you can.
- Squeezing your shoulder blades together.
- Exhale as you lift the dumbbells.
- Pause on the top.
- SLOWLY lower the weights, feeling your rear shoulders and back doing the work.
- Inhale as you lower.
- Repeat until set is complete.

Rear Raise

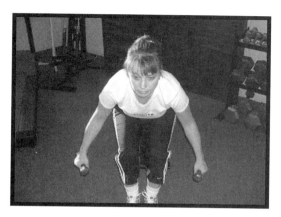

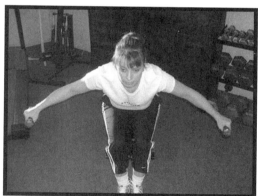

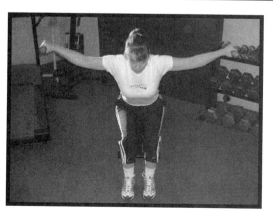

Shoulders

Side Raise

Muscles Used: Outer Shoulders
Starting Weight: 5-15 lbs.

- Standing.
- Dumbbells at your sides and palms facing each other.
- Keep elbows bent during the entire movement.
- Raise the dumbbells out to the sides like you are flying.
- Stop when the DBs are in line with or slightly above your head.
- Slowly lower, keeping elbows bent.
- Repeat until set is complete.

Shoulders

Side Raise

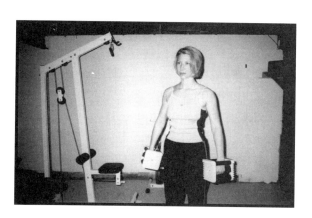

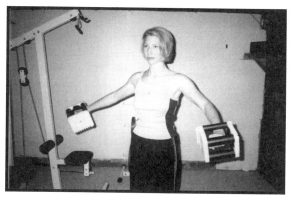

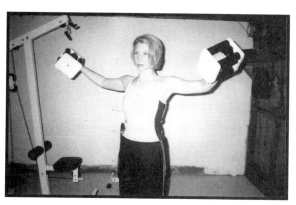

Triceps

Kickbacks

Muscles Used: Triceps
Starting Weight: 3-10 lbs.

- Grasp 2 dumbbells.
- Standing, feet shoulder width apart.
- Bend over, keeping your back flat and your head up.
- Palms facing each other.
- Bring your elbows to your sides.
- *Elbows do not move during the entire exercise.*
- Arms bent at about a 90-degree angle.
- Push the dumbbells back and up, straightening your arms.
- Pause for a second.
- FEEL your triceps flex hard at the top position.
- Exhale.
- Slowly lower to starting position keeping you head up.
- Inhale while lowering.
- Repeat until set is complete.
- TIP: To make kickbacks more effective, only lower the dumbbells about half way and then push back up. You can do this until you triceps start to fatigue and then use full range of motion on the last few reps.

Triceps
Kickbacks

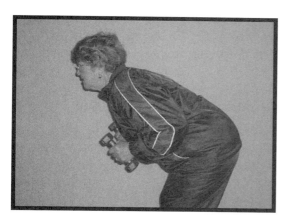

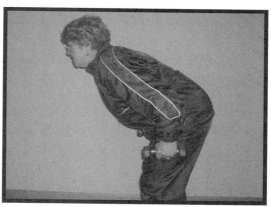

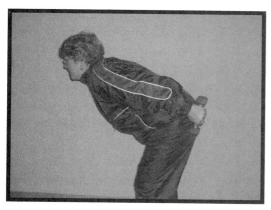

Triceps

Overhead Extensions

Muscles Used: Triceps
Starting Weight: 10-20 lbs.

- Seated, feet firmly on the floor.
- Grasp a dumbbell on the inside end with your palms flat, overlapping each other securely.
- Bring dumbbell to starting position, directly over your head.
- Elbows stay in the same position during the entire movement.
- Slowly lower the weight behind your head.
- *Keep you head up and back straight.*
- Lower as far as possible, feeling a good stretch in your triceps.
- Inhale as you lower.
- Make sure your elbows don't move.
- Push the dumbbells back up to the starting position.
- Stop right before your elbows lock out.
- Exhale as you lift the weight.
- Repeat until your set is complete.

Overhead Extensions

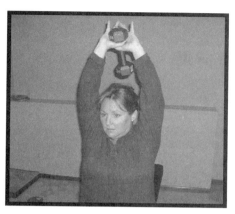

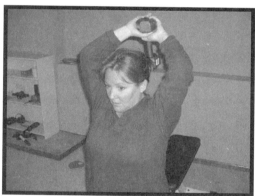

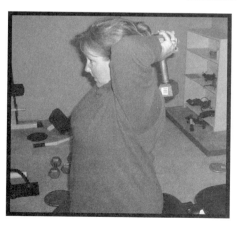

Triceps

Pushdowns

Muscles Used: Triceps
Starting Weight: 25-40 lbs.

- Stand, facing the pulldown machine, about a foot away.
- Keep your back straight, knees slightly bent and feet shoulder width apart.
- Grasp bar, palms facing down, about a foot apart.
- Pull the bar down so your elbows are touching your sides. *Then your elbows will not move during the exercise.*
- Push straight down until arms are straight.
- You should feel your triceps contract.
- Slowly resist weight until about chest height.
- Remember your elbows do not move.
- Repeat until set is complete.
- TIP: You can also use the rope attachment.

Triceps
Pushdowns

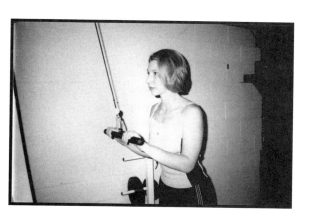

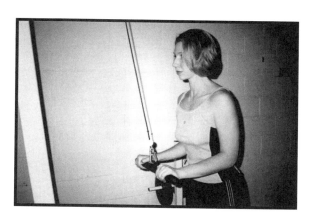

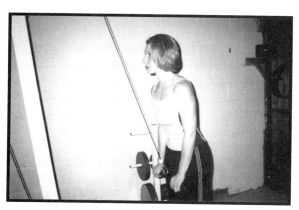

Triceps

SkullKrushers

Muscles Used: Triceps
Starting Weight: 5-15 lbs.

- Grasp 2 dumbbells.
- Lie on a bench.
- Feet firmly on the floor or bench.
- Start with the dumbbells straight over your shoulders.
- Arms straight and elbows pointed towards your feet.
- Palms facing each other.
- Elbows stay in the same position throughout exercise.
- Slowly lower the dumbbells along the sides of your head.
- Lower until you feel a good stretch in your triceps.
- Inhale as you lower.
- Pause at the bottom.
- Return to starting position.
- Stop right before your elbows lock out.
- Exhale as you lift the weights.
- Repeat until set is complete.
- TIP: Be careful not to use too heavy of dumbbells so you can not control them around your head!

SkullKrushers

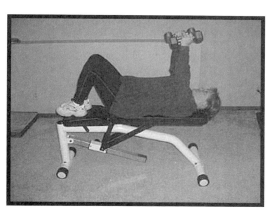

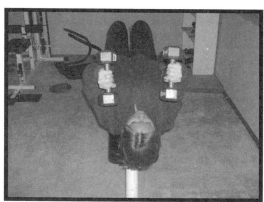

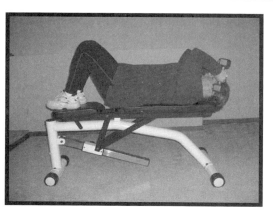

Even More Workouts that Work!

Looking to lose even more weight!?
Add more rock hard muscle!?

Books I and II are currently available.

Weight Training Workouts that Work
&
Weight Training Workouts that Work: Volume II

Plus many new workouts to download.

All are available at
www.weighttrainingworkouts.com

Questions? Need Help? Comments?
Email: james@weighttrainingworkouts.com

NEXT BOOK AVAILABLE SOON

127 Weight Training Workouts that Work

- You choose the workouts that work best for you -

About the Author

James Orvis is a personal trainer and author. For the past 15 years James has been teaching, researching, writing and using the best workouts and nutritional programs for maximum results. The goal is for anybody, any age, any fitness level, to look and feel their best! His two previous books are *Weight Training Workouts that Work* and *Weight Training Workouts that Work: Volume II*. James resides with his family in Crosslake, Minnesota.

Quick Exercise Finder